little
things

little things

A positive toolkit for when life feels stressful

FEARNE COTTON

For Laura. For showing us all true resilience.

2

Vermilion/Happy Place Books, an imprint of Ebury Publishing
20 Vauxhall Bridge Road
London SW1V 2SA

Vermilion is part of the Penguin Random House group of companies
whose addresses can be found at global.penguinrandomhouse.com

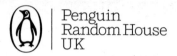

First published by Vermilion in 2024

www.penguin.co.uk

A CIP catalogue record for this book is available from the British Library

ISBN 9781785044861

Printed and bound in Great Britain by Clays Ltd, Elcograf S.p.A.

The authorised representative in the EEA is Penguin Random House Ireland,
Morrison Chambers, 32 Nassau Street, Dublin D02 YH68.

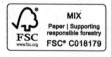

Penguin Random House is committed to a sustainable future
for our business, our readers and our planet. This book is made
from Forest Stewardship Council® certified paper

CONTENTS

INTRODUCTION

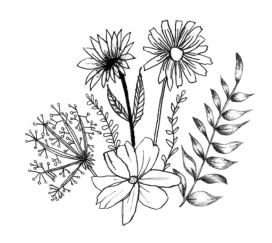

Hands up who feels stressed?

I'm pretty sure most of you raised an arm or maybe just nodded your head. And if you didn't, I'm almost certain you will have felt stressed at some point in the last couple of weeks or months. Stress is ubiquitous, and can be found in all corners of life. Often it can feel like there is a constant undercurrent of it, present when we're moving through the day. It can also crop up when we are triggered by things from the past, be it an irritating buzz of background noise or an all-consuming bombardment that blindsides us. We all feel it, yet none of us want it. Not only does it sting in the moment, but it can have a very real and long-lasting impact on our mental and physical health.

Writing this book has been a bit of an emotional roller coaster. More so than any book I've written before. The roller coaster began with an urgent ascent of enthusiasm and excitement to tackle such a huge subject. This quickly turned to worry that I wouldn't be able to do this gargantuan subject justice. That worry ironically turned to – you guessed it – stress. Reaching that point felt like a dead end and the nearest I've gotten to writer's block. This dead end led to me stepping back, reassessing how I was responding to that stress and remembering my mission.

The point of this book is not to eliminate all the stressful situations in your life – sadly, that's usually not possible, as we all suffer stress in differing ways, whether it's at work, in our relationships, with our finances, our family or in navigating all of these things. Instead, I want you to get curious about stress, notice what it is telling you and bring focus to how you respond to it.

When I have had big moments of stress, it is always the little things that help shift my perspective and stop me from drowning in it all. If we are presented with big, life-altering solutions, we often feel overwhelmed and are more likely to quit before we've even started. What we do not need in moments of stress is another thing on our list to worry about, so in this book I promise not to burden you with huge life-changing proposals. I want us all to move gently and slowly towards little changes that will help us better understand our own emotional roller coaster and be able to cope when faced with stress. I've gathered these little nuggets of advice over the years from my own lessons learned and therapies I've tried, as well as the numerous incredible conversations I have had on my podcast, *Happy Place*. I've harvested as many helpful little things as possible and have weaved them throughout these pages.

When plotting out this book my starting point was to create a map of stress. With a deep desire to get curious about the triggers around stress, I needed to have conversations that I hadn't previously had with the people I know. Strangely, I hadn't asked my friend Fran, who is an air steward, how she handles the stress of her job. I hadn't asked my friend Abbie how she copes with having a disabled son. I hadn't asked my own mum about the physical symptoms she experiences from unprocessed stress. These conversations, many of which are peppered throughout this book with their subsequent learnings, were profoundly interesting and taught me a lot. I interviewed friends and acquaintances with differing backgrounds, set-ups, living arrangements and triggers, which helped me decipher how I would divide up this book.

The five categories of stressful situations that I talk about are:

1 **Demands.** This assesses the everyday demands we face – from others, from society and the pressure we put on ourselves.

2 **Health.** Here we look at how stress directly affects our health and how health issues can themselves cause a lot of worry and stress.

3 **Control.** Whether you find comfort in controlling every step of your day, or currently feel wildly out of control, this section will explore how each end of the spectrum can lead to stress.

4 **Relationships.** Tricky dynamics, intimate relationships, friend-ships and work colleagues can cause great joy and also stress, so we will dive into managing those relationships better.

5 **Change.** Often when great change is afoot, we feel vast amounts of stress. From moving house to dealing with loss, our emotional response will often land in stress. We will also look at how stress can manifest when there isn't enough change and things become stagnant.

UNDERSTANDING STRESS

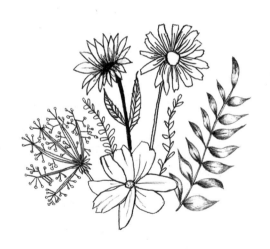

Stress appears to be more ubiquitous than ever. It may seem that way because we now talk about it more openly and understand its consequences with more clarity. Perhaps stress has always been this prevalent but previous generations felt less inclined to discuss it. Or maybe we are more stressed than ever as we attempt to keep up with the pace of modern life – every change in technology, rising prices, societal pressures, and the lack of support for those suffering.

Normalising stress is both relieving and problematic, so we need to stay on the right side of the paradox. Personally, I like to discuss stress. It can be a lonely place to assume everyone else is coping when you're not. Yet if we just sit back and accept that everyone everywhere is stressed, are we less likely to spring into action to make the little changes that can help us? We don't want to ignore the stress in our lives, but equally we don't want to acknowledge it and assume we have to put up with its relentlessness.

As Dr Gabor Maté has professed in his book *The Myth of Normal*, feeling stressed is a very normal emotional reaction to the abnormal conditions of the modern world. We are over-using technology and diluting true face-to-face human connection. We work longer hours and are not taking proper rest. We are lacking support with childcare, as the nuclear family set-up reigns in the West: where once it took a village to raise children, we are now expecting parents and single parents to cope alone. And we have an increased propensity to compare ourselves to others through social media. These are just a few examples of the many changes we have faced as humans in the last couple of decades that increase our general stress levels. All of these newer societal quirks have been normalised, but we are yet to find the appropriate coping mechanisms to deal with them.

Little Things is my attempt to collate as many supportive ideas, tools and coping modalities as possible, for my sake and yours. I am certainly not sitting here in a lotus pose professing to have all the answers to living a calmer, less stressed life. Please call my husband for clarification that I am not naturally a calm human. I jump to stress quickly, often look for the negatives and flap when it all gets too much. Just this morning my husband sent me an Instagram video of a cat climbing the walls, having been shocked by another cat. The cat was ping-ponging across the room, scratching at windowsills and running without direction. He knew it would resonate, and it did. I am often that cat when faced with stressful situations. I need this book just as much as you do.

I will work through the everyday stresses that most of us feel, but also the monumental stresses – the ones that feel colossal and very permanent. One of the reasons I am authoring this book is because I have certain stresses in my life that at times have almost derailed me, and the aftershock of those moments still echoes in corners of my life today. When it comes to big stress, I cannot make promises to extinguish those circumstances or make your life run entirely smoothly, but I hope *Little Things* becomes a comforting mate you can turn to in tricky times. This book is your safe space to express how you feel, to vent and rant, and to help you gain awareness of what is causing the stress in the first place. I hope it helps you to spot behavioural patterns when it comes to looking at how you react to stressful situations, as well as the recurring themes that make you feel stressed out.

It is important when reading the interviews within these pages not to condemn yourself for having it easier than others. Do not compare yourself to those in the book. Your stress is valid and so are your struggles. The interviews are there to give you hope, new tools and a little solace too. Each one of us experiences stress in a different way. Our triggers, reactions to stress and general coping mechanisms will all differ. Use this book to get to know yourself and your stress that bit better.

I'm also keen to not exclusively throw shade over stress, as sometimes, just sometimes, it can be a helpful response to what is going on around us. We might feel stressed before we talk in front of a group of colleagues at work. That stress could give us the adrenaline-fuelled focus we need to nail our presentation. Sometimes stress can act as a warning sign, signalling for us to make changes, get out of a situation or pivot in life. At other times it can make us stop in our tracks and reevaluate our lives and how we are behaving. See? Stress isn't entirely the bad guy.

All stress is welcome here. My aim is that we stop seeing stress as the enemy, get to know it much more intimately, and have a creative, expressive time along the way. Whenever I do deep-dive therapy, and I have done a hell of a lot of it, I learn so much about myself. If that little judgy voice is popping up again, telling you that self-exploration or self-reflection is indulgent, then silence it immediately. You are worth every bit of time and effort. Give yourself the space and time to get to know yourself better. It might feel uncomfortable at first, but through the process of reading and working through this book you might start to learn something about yourself and how you can take back control when it comes to stress.

The most empowering lesson I've learned in regard to stress over the years is knowing that we have more of a choice than we believe we do. It's not always easily practised, but having the knowledge is a great start. When we feel stressed, we tend to react rather than respond. When we react, we don't give ourselves time to pause and think clearly. We let emotions and past experiences inform how we react and often fall into negative habitual patterns of behaviour. Instead, we can choose to respond. Responding requires a thoughtful pause, a moment of awareness and a considered choice that will better serve us.

I'm not here to extinguish all stress, or to tell you simply to 'stress less' about something that's causing you harm, but I do believe the little things in this book will give you a neat toolkit you can rely on when things feel too much.

Right, are you ready to get stuck into stress? I promise we'll go as slow and gently as possible. It'll be interesting, explorative and potentially quite fun. Expect honesty, storytelling, moments for you to reflect and hopefully a sigh of relief as we all attempt to understand stress a little better together.

AN EXPERT LOOK AT STRESS

To examine stress thoroughly I thought we would kick off with a few deep-dive chats with some great minds who know their onions, starting with Dr Jud Brewer, a psychiatrist, bestselling author and thought leader who specialises in habit change and the science of self-mastery. He has spent years studying the habits we form, often in times of stress, and how we can use mindfulness to help with creating new thought patterns and behaviours. I'm keen to learn more about what is going on mentally, physically and emotionally when we experience stress.

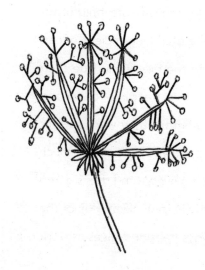

Interview with Dr Jud Brewer

Dr Jud, obviously we know that there have been very challenging times throughout history and that certain communities during these times will have endured huge amounts of stress. Do you believe we are collectively more stressed now than ever before?

DJ: In the modern world there are a lot more things to be aware of, and we need to get a good balance of what information is helpful for survival and what is not. There is disinformation and misinformation out there, which can lead to overwhelm. Our fear mechanisms are helpful for survival but can also be very unhelpful. Our ancient ancestors might have heard rustling in the bushes outside their dwellings which would lead to them needing to go and retrieve information to gather whether they were safe or not. That information is helpful, but if you look at how much information there is today, knowing everything that's going on in the world, it's not necessarily helpful. Seeing all of the bad news out there doesn't always help and gives us a lot of anxiety for the future. That overwhelm and stress turns into anxiety. That anxiety can then turn into fear and dread for the future. We are so used to looking into the future.

What is the difference between stress and anxiety?

The biggest difference is that stress has a clear object or precipitant, while anxiety doesn't necessarily have one. Anxiety is a feeling of nervousness about an event or time in the future.

How is stress impacting the physical body?

It's hard to quantify but the consensus is that the mind and body are connected, and that stress has a big impact on the physical body, but it is also reciprocal. If we are enduring physical stress, we are then more susceptible to mental stress. There is no clear physiological benefit of experiencing anxiety in the short term or the long term: it can raise blood pressure and it can cause cardiac issues, as well as a host of other problems. The reciprocal relationship between the body and mind is significant and we are still early on in our studies as to how badly the body is affected by mental stress and vice versa. I don't think the details of how stress affects the body are important: we know it's bad and that's all we need to know.

We will all experience stress in our lives, but how we cope with it will differ. Do you think our coping mechanisms are purely down to where and how we grew up?

I don't think it's that simple. It can certainly influence our conditioning. The modelling from our parents absolutely affects us; yet some people are just born chilled out and that could be down to our genes, and we have no control over our genes. What's important to remember is that we do have control over our minds, and that's where we can really start to see the results of the moments where we are reacting vs responding to stress. We can train our brains to get in the habit of responding to stress differently.

When we are stressed, one way we might react to that stress is to fall into bad habits. We don't make the best choices and bad habits usually equal a quick fix of pleasure. How do we begin to break bad habits, so we respond rather than react to stress?

We found in our studies that there is a three-step process for behavioural change. The first step is being able to recognise what the habitual behaviour is. The moments where we are turning to social media, alcohol or where we get into a bad habit loop of worrying; whatever behaviour distracts us and makes us feel like we are in control. So, acknowledge these actions; if you're on autopilot you might not even be aware of your reactions.

The second step is to hack the brain and understand that the only way to change habits is through adjusting the reward value of a behaviour. We might assume that once we spot a bad habit we can just choose to stop doing it, but it doesn't really work like that. Willpower alone won't work. It's not how our brain operates. Willpower is more myth than muscle. Neuroscience tells us the brain wants to do things that are rewarding. We have to ask ourselves a simple question: 'What am I getting from this?' We have to drop in and see how rewarding the experience actually is.

If it's not rewarding, we are going to become disenchanted and then step out of the process of doing it. Using an app, we studied overeaters and saw how quickly the reward value changed when we asked participants to focus on how rewarding the experience was. We found that it only takes 10–15 times for someone paying attention when they over-eat for the reward value to drop below zero. It doesn't take a lot of time; it takes awareness. It's the same with worrying. You start to become aware that the worrying is doing nothing for you. It's a critical step, as you have to become disenchanted with the bad habit once you see how unrewarding the behaviour is. You need a better offering, but it can't be a substitute. For example, you don't want to substitute candy for cigarettes. You have to find something that is intrinsically rewarding. You can bring curiosity to a craving and instantly notice which feeling is better. Worrying or curiosity? When you get curious you start to see that the cravings are just physical sensations and thoughts. When you are curious about a feeling or behaviour, the change part of the process is almost effortless, as awareness becomes the magic pill.

Neuroplasticity [the brain's ability to form new connections through learning and other experiences] is deeply empowering, as each time you make a positive change you feel encouraged to do it again. Some of this is also surely about discomfort? It seems we are all becoming increasingly allergic to discomfort, but my belief is it's imperative to sit with discomfort to move through loops of bad habit. Is this correct, Dr Jud?

I agree. I think in today's world we are more and more habituated to this narrative that we should never be uncomfortable. Take a pill, use a distraction, et cetera. Even if you're at the traffic lights you see people's laps glowing as heads are craned down towards phones, as collectively we can't even deal with a three-second wait for the lights to change. That's the level of distress tolerance that we now lack. That's now being modelled to kids, which is not good.

I had a patient who came in and told me his head was going to explode if he didn't have a cigarette. I used a whiteboard and a marker and diagrammed what it felt like for him. We created a graph which illustrated how his craving grew and grew and then crested and dived back down. The patient looked at the graph and realised that, at the crest of the craving, he always smoked, but that he didn't have to as the craving peaked then troughed naturally. He had just never waited long enough to find that out.

How does mindfulness weave its way into the conversation of stress reduction?

The short answer is that if you look at that three-step process we talked about earlier, you can see it in play. I think of mindfulness as awareness, but alongside curiosity. You have to be aware if you're in a habit loop – you've got to be aware of what the results are – but you also have to be curious about that awareness. The curiosity helps us just be rather than constantly do.

Yes, it seems we need to see how short-term discomfort could stop us from experiencing long-term agony and more stress, perhaps.

Yes, but I have to bring up what's known as 'delay discounting' here. The further away the long-term detriments are, the less likely we are to do something about it. If it's too far away to be a driving force, then little action will be taken. The craving in the now is stronger than the worry about the long term. That's why we have to tackle behaviour in the now rather than the future. This is how we create positive change.

Meditation is a big part of your life and it's known to help people when it comes to stress reduction. How does it help us?

I think meditation itself helps us have a dedicated time to practise mapping out how our minds work. We can start to notice our own behaviour around stress and quieten our surrounding noise, so we can look internally more clearly. It is one supportive way of becoming more aware. Informal practices are often equally as powerful as meditation. Whatever piques your curious awareness is enough. You can even just practise being aware of your surroundings for a few moments, but do so regularly throughout the day.

I guess that could also lead to other benefits, such as experiencing awe. We sometimes bypass awe, as we are rushing about and in habit loops.

Yes, I like to think of awe as openness, whereas stress and anxiety feel closed. You cannot be closed and open at the same time. It's a binary contradiction, so look for what helps you feel open as it will be a lot harder to be stressed out in those times.

One of my big goals while writing *Little Things* has been to explore the difference between stress and anxiety. At times in my own life, I have found it hard to see where stress ends and anxiety begins, as they've felt inextricable from one another. Dr Jud's explanation has unpicked the psychology and allows us to differentiate between the two. As a recap: stress has a clear precipitant whereas anxiety doesn't. To get even more granular, this means that when we are stressed, we can clearly notice the situation, person or problem that is causing the emotion, whereas with anxiety the catalyst may be untethered and unrelated to one specific and acute cause. Knowing this gives us a better chance of finding the little things that can help reduce both. If we know the causes of our stress, we can dissect them and potentially make changes to the situation or our response to them. We may notice our anxiety naturally and subsequently lessening. We may also have the ability to get clearer on why we feel anxious.

I love that Dr Jud also spoke about that feeling of openness. Maybe you have experienced it while looking at the undulating sea, or when gazing at the night stars? It certainly feels a lot nicer than feeling closed and restricted. Think about something that makes you feel that way. I feel closed when I think about overwhelm, gossip and unkindness. It's a clear way to distinguish the difference between curiosity and stress. Curiosity is an openness, a willingness to explore, whereas stress is a dead end with little room for movement. It's a brilliant way to bring the physical body into the equation, too. When I feel openness, I feel relaxed, comfortable and alive; whereas when I feel closed, I feel tense, uncomfortable and lethargic.

understanding stress

Throughout the rest of your day today, or tomorrow, come back to this page and note how many times you felt closed versus open. Write down what causes you to feel both.

OPEN   CLOSED

Interview with Owen O'Kane

Someone who knows a thing or two about managing stress is my good friend Owen O'Kane. As a psychotherapist, speaker and bestselling author of books *Ten to Zen* and *How to Be Your Own Therapist*, he has a lot to share on the subject. I have not only collaborated with Owen professionally, I've also worked with him to help understand my own thought patterns and responses to stress. What I've learned from Owen has changed my life and given me a lot more mental peace, so I was keen for him to share some of his advice here.

Owen, do you see themes in the causes of stress in your patients? Are there common themes that are universal?

OO: Despite the uniqueness of people's stories, I do see themes that are common in the causes of stress. These tend to fall into four categories and I believe they are universal, especially in western society:

People generally struggle with the uncertainty and unpredictability of everyday life and its challenges. If anxiety is an intolerance of uncertainty, then we are an anxious, stressed population. But my preference is not to label this diagnostically: rather, I like to view this through the lens of humanity. To be human is to sometimes struggle.

1 Many people are overwhelmed with the volume of life's demands and don't find a balance that enables them to cope better.

2 We live in a world that is increasingly busy, noisy, polluted, divided, threatened, discontented, virtual and disconnected. This is creating an experience of destabilisation.

3 The human mind is 'hard wired' to be vigilant for threat, which is the healthy side of stress. That said, it is not equipped to be on high alert all the time, which many people are.

Do you think we collectively underestimate the physical impact stress has on us?

Unquestionably, yes. Neuroscience, modern medicine and psychology inform us that prolonged or chronic periods of stress have a detrimental impact on physical health.

We cannot separate mind and body; they are interlinked. There is always two-way communication between both. If the mind is depleted or struggling to function well, then it will communicate that clearly to the body. Consequently, a highly stressed mind will mirror in the body through illness.

I think of this as nature's way of trying to force someone to stop, slow down or reregulate. Mind and body are in a constant state of trying to find a place of balance and equilibrium. Of course, the same is true during periods of illness or physical neglect, when the body communicates with the mind in the same way. There are constant feedback loops of communication between both worlds. Learning to listen and work with both is crucial.

Why do some of us cope better with stress than others?

Some traditional research links 'coping well' with two personality types: Type A and Type B personalities. It is thought that Type A personalities are more likely to be predisposed to stress than their counterparts, Type B. While this makes sense to a point, I don't entirely agree.

I believe the reasons why some people cope better are more varied and complex. In my experience there is never a single factor. People come with a story. That story may include negative experiences such as adversity, trauma, deprivation, family dysfunction, poverty, crime, sociological factors, cultural norms and learned experiences. The list is endless. It is also worth remembering that someone's ability to cope isn't a linear process. It may change during certain periods in life, for example with bereavement, loss or any period of major transition.

I think we need more focus and research on the 'how' we can help people cope rather than the 'why' they aren't coping. People aren't one thing or the other. We will never have a definitive answer to the question of why. But we can find breakthroughs in helping people move forward.

What do you believe is the difference between stress and anxiety?

For me this is almost like the 'you say tomato, I say tomato' thing. Sometimes it's just linguistics.

Stress itself isn't considered a mental health disorder under *DSM* [*Diagnostic and Statistical Manual of Mental Disorders*, the principal guide to psychiatric disorders used in the US] guidelines. That said, acute stress disorder is. This is said to be linked to specific fear behaviour after a traumatic event.

Anxiety disorders can fall into several categories: for example, generalised anxiety disorder, social anxiety, health anxiety, OCD and so on.

I believe we need to focus less on pathologising people with labels that include the word 'disorder'. You are not disordered if you are stressed or anxious. Likewise, I don't think it matters too much whether stress causes anxiety or vice versa. My interest is human distress.

To be human means that sometimes we will all struggle. There will be times when the human mind will work harder than it needs to and enter a hypervigilant, protective state. Yes, it's trying to help and protect us! When we realise that, we can begin to negotiate with the mind and learn ways of quieting the noise and functioning better. It's really quite simple. But I do appreciate it takes time and practice.

What can stress teach us about ourselves?

I think the message of stress is clear and it doesn't need to be overly complicated. Stress is an internal barometer that is communicating to you that you are not in a state of balance. Every person's responsibility is to listen to that message and find their way back. Sometimes support and help will be needed. But there is always a way back.

Here are some other things I think are worth bearing in mind when we look at stress.

❀ The links between self-compassion and stress. How we treat and talk to ourselves is everything. Techniques don't work if your self-talk is unkind or critical.

❀ When you see stress as an ally, not the enemy, everything changes.

❀ Diet, lifestyle, food, and everyday boundaries can't be ignored or excluded when managing stress. They are the essential foundation of wellness.

❀ To be connected to others in a time of stress is a must. Loneliness and disconnection feed stress.

As Owen says, the physical body usually responds when we are mentally stressed, and we will dive into this further in the Health section of the book. I love the idea that we can learn to listen to the body and see stress as an indicator that we are out of balance. I'm also glad that Owen brought up the need to talk to yourself kindly. Negative self-talk is a bad habit that most of us are in, but we often don't realise how damaging it is. While we work through the different themes and exercises in the book, bear in mind the tone of voice you use towards yourself. Are you in the habit of being your own worst critic? Keep coming back to those questions as we explore stress.

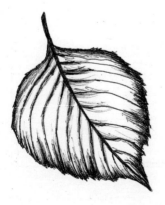

YOUR STRESS PROFILE

It's time to look at what is causing you stress.

Write a list as long or short as needed about everything you are currently stressed about. Go for it, be unfiltered. This is your space.

I AM STRESSED ABOUT ...

Now let's get even more curious and look at what else is going on. With each of the situations, people or memories that you have listed that cause you stress, sit for a moment and think about whether you believe you *react* or *respond* to the stress. Do any of the stress triggers cause you to act in a habitual way? Are you in the habit of blaming others? Turning on yourself? Hiding? Drinking too much? There is no judgement here. We all have our coping mechanisms. This part of the book is a chance to really assess if our current coping mechanisms are working for us or not.

How do you react to stress?

It's not an easy exercise, as we have to get very real with ourselves and admit that, at times, we are letting habit rule. It can feel humbling, scary and shameful to admit how we react to stress, but that's all very normal. I will not allow you to even consider slipping into self-loathing at this stage – judging yourself will not help at all. Know that we are all in this together. When you feel ready, have a look at whether any of your current coping mechanisms actually work for you. If they do, great. If they don't, then let's make some little changes together.

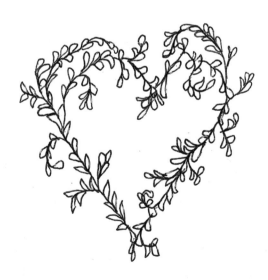

DEMANDS

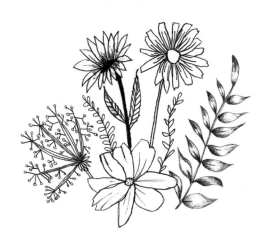

Life is full of demands and often there is not much we can do about it. Whether we have families, jobs, social circles, pets or people we care for, we will be aware of the demands that pull us in every direction. Some of these demands fit into our routines; they are less obvious as they are woven into the rhythm of our daily lives. Some are thoroughly enjoyable, as we feel boosted when helping out or being of service. But others feel draining, impossible and extremely stressful. Many of these demands will be immovable. If you feel stressed because the demands of caring for a sick parent are tipping you over the edge, you cannot eradicate that demand. Or if your toddler's needs are causing you stress, you cannot simply mitigate those either.

The aim of this chapter is not to rid ourselves of all responsibility, but to find ways to lessen our reaction to pressures in our lives and develop coping strategies to get us through busy, stressful times. When we have awareness of how the stress feels, where it lands in our bodies and how we respond to it, we can spot patterns and then start to make decisions that help to get us through it.

I've wasted a lot of time wishing certain elements of my life were easier without noticing what I've learned from those challenges and how much more resilient I am because of them. With that in mind, in this chapter I will not be advising that any of us drop all of the demands we face in order to enjoy a life of pure comfort and ease, but instead see what we can learn from our challenges.

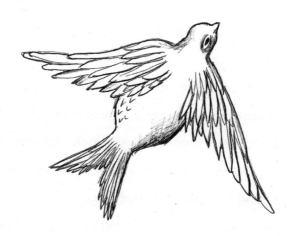

OVERWHELM

Depending on where we are at in our lives and our age and set-up, the length of our list of demands will differ. I noticed a big shift in life when I became a stepmum, as I went from exclusively dealing with work demands to having family ones too. At 29 I became a stepmum to Arthur and Lola, and at 31 I became mother to Rex. I got married at 32 and then had another child, Honey, at 34. These are precious moments I am beyond grateful for, but we rarely talk openly about the demands that come along with such joy, in fear of judgement. Having kids in whatever capacity, or a partner in your life, means you must consciously divide your time, headspace, and choices to facilitate others. Often those with kids or partners feel they cannot speak out about the pressures they feel as there is a sense that you should exclusively feel gratitude. This book is a judgement-free zone. We don't have time for guilt or worry as to what others might think. We cannot sideline our own wellbeing because we have certain boxes ticked and should just be grateful for our lot. There are parts of life that can be glorious and gratifying, yet still feel stressful. Let's not be afraid to admit that. If there is stress, let's talk about it, dig about in it, and help each other out.

My working life has also expanded in ways that I could not have imagined, which is bloody glorious yet also presents many demands. Although I have established that this is a judgement-free zone I do feel a disclaimer coming on: I love my job, I feel insanely lucky that I get to express myself in my working life, I feel privileged to be able to write books, interview incredible people and put festivals on, yet ... stress is inevitable in most jobs, even very enjoyable ones. The public nature of my job, and the fact that multiple projects are in the works at any one time, add greater demands. It's a pressure I thrive on, but one that also leads to insomnia and physical stress if I am not looking after myself properly.

When we don't have the headspace to notice how much the demands of life are stressing us out, we end up at overwhelm. I have noticed over the last three or four years that my overwhelm is very cyclical. It usually starts with an insecurity that I am not doing enough. I then pile on the work projects, offer to help out on school trips, say yes to all social events, then hit overwhelm. I know this cycle well, yet I haven't managed to break it. When I hit overwhelm, I panic. Rather than calmly telling those around me that I cannot facilitate all that I have promised, I start to panic that I will be hated and rejected, so I push myself to exhaustion.

On a scale of 1–10, how overwhelmed do you feel at the moment?

....

Do you often say yes to doing more, helping out more, even when you know it'll probably lead to overwhelm?

....

....

....

Is your overwhelm cyclical, or do you notice certain times of the year or changes in your mood or general wellbeing that lead you to it?

....

....

....

....

Little things to help with overwhelm

❊ **When I feel overwhelmed** I will go for a walk. Trainers on, gentle music in my headphones, and I walk. There is something about the forward motion of a walk that feels like you are moving emotional baggage on.

❊ **I've recently become very interested in sound therapy** and have found it very cathartic. Either during a workout or just alone in my home, I use sound to move on tension in my body. I either shout or groan loudly on an exhale and let anger, stress and pent-up anxiety out of my body. It's also incredible for your throat. I have had throat issues due to stress over the years, which have shown up as a tightened throat and, at its worst, a throat cyst, which is not ideal in my job, so I use this technique regularly. You may feel self-conscious at first, but when you get into the swing of it and feel the benefits there will be no holding you back. You don't need to overanalyse the emotions that arise: just let out the sound. Sound is energy, so you are quite literally helping stuck energy to move on. RAAAR!

❀ **Shaking your body** is another amazing way to release stress from the body. Animals do this after they have experienced something stressful. There is no right way to do this, just shake your whole body either all at once or concentrate on areas where you feel you might need to release tension. Do it to music or just in silence.

❀ **Give yourself a hug.** This is technically a yoga move and probably my favourite one. Wrap your arms around yourself and hold your own body. Not only does it feel like a nice stretch, but also your body signals to your brain that you are safe. When you need a good hug, don't forget about giving yourself one.

❀ **Breathe.** It's obvious, and something we do all day, but I always find if I concentrate on my breath my body reacts well. My heart stops racing, my muscles feel less tense and my thoughts slow down. You can count your breaths if that helps you hold focus, or imagine your lungs filling up and then deflating again. There are loads of lovely breathwork practices on our Happy Place app you might want to try. Always breathe before you react to stress.

little things

Notice how much you are taking on. If you need to let someone down for your own mental and physical wellbeing, then be honest with them. If they are a good mate they will understand. If you can delegate or leave less important demands until later down the line to give yourself a breather, then you'll find tiny pockets within your day to practise any of the above. If you have trouble saying no, we will get stuck into boundaries later on in this section of the book.

demands

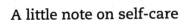

A little note on self-care

Self-care is an overused phrase that has almost lost its meaning, as we see it splashed across memes and TikTok videos, but it's an important topic to focus on. If we aren't taking care of ourselves, we cannot take care of others. If we aren't giving ourselves love and time, then we cannot do the same for others. It doesn't have to be grand, particularly luxurious or time-consuming, but it does make a huge difference.

When was the last time you did something just for you – a hot bath, a walk in the park, or watching your favourite film in your pyjamas?

....

....

If you are struggling to remember when you last did something nice for yourself, this is your chance. I will happily give you permission to carve that time out as soon as you can. I often need enormous amounts of prompting to do so, but I always feel better afterwards and much less overwhelmed and stressed.

PRESSURE

As teenagers we might get our first taste of proper stress from the demands of life with the onset of exams. As parents of teenagers, we may worry about our children experiencing pressure and feel a little helpless. At the time of writing this book my stepson has just finished university and my stepdaughter is sitting her A level exams; huge life moments that feel very defining. Over the years I have done many talks in secondary schools on this very subject and always try to remind the students and parents that bad exam results are not the end of the road.

We are led to believe that satisfactory results are life-defining, yet while they can offer certain opportunities, I don't believe it's helpful to have that immense pressure to perform on one specific day. Attaining good exam results to ensure a 'good job' seems to get conflated with our general future happiness. If you pass all of your exams, that may lead to a job offer, but this doesn't guarantee happiness. Equally, if you fail your exams, or get results lower than expected, your long-term happiness won't be affected. Yes, there will be disappointment, and you might have to change your plans, but it's not the end of the road. There are always other options and opportunities to think outside of the box. Sometimes getting straight out into a work environment is just as beneficial as going to university. Even applying for work experience and making valuable contacts in your chosen field will make a big impact on your future options.

Remembering that good exam results don't impact your long-term happiness may not take all of the heat off, but it might lessen the stress ever so slightly. I have interviewed countless people who found jobs they love and thrive in after failing exams, or leaving education prematurely. My dear friend Elizabeth Day does a bloody good job of promoting the benefits of failing in her podcast *How to Fail*. Give it a listen for some incredibly inspirational stories.

What have you learned from failing? Can you think back to a time where things didn't quite go to plan? What did you learn from that experience?

....

....

....

....

If you, or your child, are feeling stressed due to revision or exams, can you list one thing you could do today that could help lessen the stress?

A little note on neurodivergence

If you are neurodivergent, or have a child who is, your concerns or struggles may be more complex, making the demands feel heavier and the stress that accompanies it more tense. Even more reason to think outside the box and play to your strengths in whatever shape they take. I've interviewed many people who have ADHD, ASD, OCD, and dyslexia, and I have learned so much in discussing their paths in life and how they have used their neurodivergence to their benefit. I also have people in my life who are neurodivergent, which has taught me a hell of a lot. The more we learn about neurodivergence collectively, the more we understand the strengths and brilliance of the symptoms rather than seeing them as a hindrance or problematic.

Little things to reduce pressure

❀ **Make a schedule for yourself to work to.** It could be a colour-coded list, sticky notes, or a spreadsheet.

❀ **Plan together with your child to go for a walk to create small breaks amongst the revision.** Even a twenty-minute walk could help reset the nervous system, so you both feel less stressed and physically less tense.

❀ **Wake up an hour earlier and finish revising earlier.** Having time at the end of the day to properly unwind can aid better sleep and lessen stress.

Often it's the tiny, incremental steps that help lessen the stress rather than huge changes: the little things.

PERSPECTIVE

A few years ago, I interviewed one of my favourite authors, Elizabeth Gilbert. She had not long before our chat experienced losing her girlfriend, Rayya, to cancer. We talked about the pain and heartache of bereavement but also how her perspective changed hugely during that time. On one occasion, as she sat by Rayya's bedside, her inbox offered up some newfound clarity. Knowing that somebody she loved so much would soon leave her highlighted that their bond was more important than most of her worries. She took out her phone, looked at the stress-inducing, bulging inbox of emails from people she knew, half knew, and really didn't know, and deleted every single one. This may seem like an extreme move and one that you're not prepared to sign up for, but it does exhibit how we can reframe what is stressful to us and why.

Can you think back to a stressful time and how your priorities and perspective may have changed?

....

....

Little things to help with perspective

When I'm struggling with finding perspective, I like to do what I call the 'zoom out'. I picture myself sitting on the sofa in my home, then, as if a small drone camera were focused on me, I zoom out. I pull focus to an aerial view of my house as a tiny dot in the town I live in. Then I zoom out further to see the whole of the UK, in the blue of the sea. Then I pull focus to see the entirety of planet Earth floating in space. Then further out so that Earth becomes a small rock in the gargantuan universe. Then out again until our galaxy is a swirling mass of light.

Does it really matter that I haven't emailed someone back? Or that I forgot to pack my son's sports kit? Does it matter so much that I haven't washed my hair in five days and I ate cereal for dinner? My little stresses and worries seem even smaller when I zoom the hell out.

ONE AT A TIME

I think about Elizabeth Gilbert and her empty inbox a lot as I personally find a string of unanswered messages highly stressful. One look at my inbox can cause the muscles around my shoulder blades to tense up, and my jaw to tighten into stone. If I really break it down, the demand I feel from my inbox is an accumulated stress. Each email on its own is doable. The individual emails themselves are hopefully low-stress in content. It's the accumulation of emails that feels heavy on my shoulders, and the accumulation of outside stress on top of that. When I am cooking for my kids, cleaning the kitchen up, texting mates back and worrying about these emails, I lose the plot altogether. I do not think rationally in these moments and end up irritable and snappy. My husband and kids don't deserve the overspill of stress, so I try to compartmentalise where the demands are coming from and park those that are lower down the priority list. Will the world end if I don't reply on the same day? I highly doubt it.

Little things for organising chaos

Below, list the demands that are on your shoulders at the moment, in order of urgency. Number 1 is your priority, going right down to number 10, which is the lowest in importance on your list. Give yourself a break today and do not give anything above number 5 any brain space.

1 ....

2 ....

3 ....

4 ....

5 ....

6 ....

7 ....

8 ....

9 ....

10 ....

BOUNDARIES

We are not superhuman and cannot do everything on our lists in one day. Also, we sometimes have to let others down. Maybe we had promised to meet a friend socially or had offered a favour with a work project which we now don't feel capable of completing. I always attempt to stick to my promises, but if my stress levels are high and the demands of life feel too much, I will approach the situation honestly and hope for understanding. Setting boundaries is key when it comes to reducing stress. First, we need to have a clear understanding of how much we can take on. Have you already got a lot on your plate or is there room to help others out and meet others' needs? Only you will know the answer to this and who you genuinely want to help. Once you acknowledge how thinly you're spreading yourself, start to cut back on spending time with those who drain you and say no to demands from those you don't have the time or energy to help. If you are reading this and happen to be British, you will know that blurting out an apology for almost anything comes extremely naturally. When setting boundaries, it is of paramount importance that you do not over-explain or apologise too much. I have to tell myself this every time I set a boundary.

I end up rewriting texts and emails, deleting the word 'sorry' many times before pressing send. A firm, short answer is sufficient. Below, write out the boundary you would like to set with someone in your life. If you find yourself over-explaining, cross out your statement or request and start over. Do this as many times as you need to. You can also practise saying it aloud if you will be speaking directly to the other person.

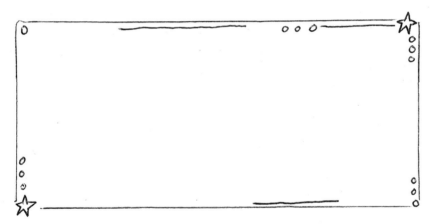

Most good eggs out there will meet your boundary with understanding. Perhaps you can't look after your neighbour's dog as arranged next week because your work commitments have increased, and you know you are going to feel even more stressed and overwhelmed. When you tell your neighbour, the likelihood is that they will respond with empathy and understanding.

Boundary crosser

So, what if your boundary is met with hostility or anger? This is the part where you must not catch the guilt. The other person's reaction is not your responsibility. Sitting in the discomfort after telling someone 'no' or setting a boundary can be tough. I worked with someone who was incredibly demanding and spoke with such authority that I usually ended up acquiescing and meeting their needs. At this point in my life, I didn't have the time, knowledge or energy to set proper boundaries, which is something I now regret. I hadn't built up the confidence to explain that I was unable to meet their demands, so I usually gave this person what they needed, then felt huge doses of resentment afterwards. You've guessed it: this working relationship did not end well. One fiery argument and it was over. I built up the confidence to say no for the first time and they walked. As I said, none of this stuff is easy, but my God I learned so much.

I recently read Melissa Urban's bestselling book about boundaries, and it felt like I was learning a new language. I couldn't believe it was possible to tell someone no, or to tell others what you needed, on a daily basis. I had always reserved setting boundaries for emergency situations. *The Book of Boundaries* even offers up scripts you can use in various situations to assist you on your journey.

Little things to help set a boundary

Think of all the moments this week where you said yes but really meant no. How many of those yeses should have been noes?

If your boundary is met with a lack of understanding, anger or upset, try not to react in the moment. If you are creating a boundary for the right reasons, then quietly go back to remembering why you set it in the first place. You may need to reconfirm your boundary or give the other person time to process what you've said. When you start setting boundaries for the first time, sometimes other people don't react well, as they are used to you being available, or simply saying yes. Remember that their reaction is their responsibility.

If you find setting boundaries uncomfortable, know that this short-term discomfort is preferable to the long-term discomfort of doing things you don't actually want to do. It might not be instantly easy but in the long run it's a worthwhile switch-up.

Helping others

Helping others is a gift and proven to be one of the best things you can do to increase your own happiness, but it has to work for you and fit around the other demands in your life. To stop stress creeping in you need to be aware of when helping becomes martyrdom.

On the next page, write a list of the people, organisations or causes you help. It can include your kids, family members, colleagues, mates, charities, and so on. Next to each, write if it causes you stress, joy, or maybe a bit of both. Once you've completed the list, have a think about whether you need to set some new boundaries or have some honest conversations with those dynamics that feel stressful. Who is asking too much of you? Who have you not been clear with about what you can and cannot offer?

People-pleasing

If I were to look back on some of my most stressful moments, they would more than likely be due to people-pleasing. People-pleasing is a direct result of having very few boundaries in place. If you relate to any of the below pointers, you are more than likely a people-pleaser.

- ❀ You say yes when you mean no.
- ❀ You take care of everyone but yourself.
- ❀ You judge yourself harshly.
- ❀ You fear rejection.
- ❀ You're overly responsible.
- ❀ You often stay quiet and don't voice your opinion.
- ❀ You often feel exhausted.

MY COMMITMENTS

1 ....

2 ....

3 ....

4 ....

5 ....

6 ....

7 ....

8 ....

I tick enough pointers on the list to 100% classify as a people-pleaser. If you do too, you'll know that it usually always comes with stress. You feel overstretched, discombobulated, and spun out. It is not easy to unpick all of the learned behaviour of being a people-pleaser, but it's not impossible. My promise at the start of the book was not to overburden any of us and to give us little things to help instead. So this week, see if you can manage saying no or putting yourself first. Just try it once this week and see how it feels. It may feel uncomfortable and alien at first, but over time, with practice, we can make it a positive habit that reduces stress. Come back to this page after you tried out saying no, or putting yourself first, and write a little about how it made you feel.

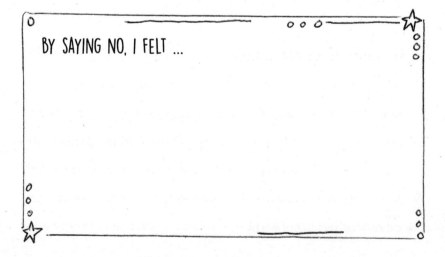

BY SAYING NO, I FELT …

Little things to help you say no

❀ 'Thank you so much for thinking of me. At the moment I am trying to take more time out for my general wellbeing, so I won't be coming along.'

❀ 'Sadly I won't be able to help out this time, but best of luck with it all.'

❀ 'Sounds like it's going to be a really great event/party/dinner but I won't be coming along as life is very busy at the moment and I don't have the bandwidth.'

Feel free to make these more personal to you and the situation but remember to not over-explain or apologise.

When boundaries are ignored

It's one thing to set a boundary but that doesn't mean it will be listened to or respected. If your boundary is ignored you have every right to restate it. If your boundaries are further ignored you may have to have a difficult conversation or lose that person from your life altogether. All the while we have to remember we cannot change how others act. If we have persistently set a boundary which is ignored, we might need to find some acceptance. Finding acceptance doesn't mean letting the other person off the hook, it means allowing yourself some mental peace. Keeping contact with that person to a minimum and accepting that you cannot change them will give you more mental freedom.

Acceptance doesn't have to be instant. It might be something you cultivate over time. Do you feel it's possible to have acceptance over the demands you cannot change?

....

....

....

Little things to help you feel less guilty

Next time you are confronted with a new demand that you do not feel you can cope with, you could:

❀ **Take a deep breath, steady yourself and don't rush.**

❀ **If things feel scary, or deeply uncomfortable, remember that this is normal.** It might also be a new concept for the other person involved to hear the word no.

❀ **Remember you have every right to express what you believe is right for you** and that the other person's reaction is not your responsibility. As a friend once said to me: 'don't catch the guilt'.

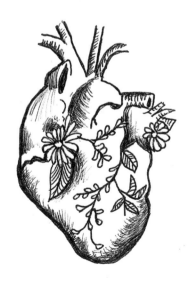

THE PILLARS

On those magical days where things are running smoothly, where I've had eight delicious hours of sleep the night before, my kids made it to school on time and I'm on top of my to-do list, I feel boosted by the demands that lie ahead. On a bad day it will only take one email I wasn't expecting to tip me over the edge. Sometimes it's not the amount or flavour of demand that's the problem; it's our state of mind. If you stub your toe on a good day, you'll whisper *ouch* and keeping walking. If you stub your toe on a dreadful day, you're likely to fall to the floor and whimper about how everything is going wrong. Dr Julie Smith, author of the bestselling book *Why Has Nobody Told Me This Before?*, recently told me on my *Happy Place* podcast that we have five basics that need to be in balance for us to keep on track with our mental health.

1 Diet (i.e. what you are eating)
2 Sleep
3 Exercise
4 Routine
5 Social contact

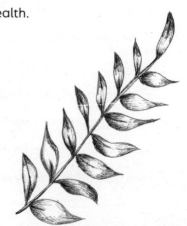

If one of those is slightly out of balance, we can easily feel like we cannot cope. What if you work nights, have a small nocturnal baby, or are poorly and have no appetite now? Sometimes the basics are knocked and it's out of our control, but in these moments we need to take a closer look at what we can control and how we can boost the other areas. If, for example, you are seriously lacking a good night's sleep due to young children or shift work, then it's even more important that you make sure you're eating as well as you can and checking in with mates when you feel low and tired. If you cannot exercise due to ill health or long work hours, ensure you are getting the right amount of sleep – not too much, not too little – and keep an eye on your routine.

Dr Julie went on to explain that we need routine but it's also important for us to leave room for spontaneity and adventure. I am the sort of person who feels very safe when I am in a routine, but I have to be careful not to block myself from experiences that could benefit me. My love of routine can make me a bit of a hermit, especially in the winter, so I really have to check in with how much I'm exposing myself to new experiences. My husband and I have organised a babysitter tonight so we can go for dinner for the first time in months and, as I sit here typing, I'm already working out how to get out of it so I can go to bed early and read. I want to spend time with my husband and know how important it is for us to carve out time for one another, yet I'm anxious that I'll be shattered tomorrow. Tonight is the perfect example of a moment where it is healthy to break free of my routine and leave space for fun, time out and a new experience.

Little things to help get the balance back

Below, under each heading, note down if you think you're in balance or not in each area. Don't beat yourself up if you aren't eating well right now, or not exercising much, or going through a bad patch of sleep: just notice where there is room for movement.

❀ **Diet.** Did you eat nutritious food today?

....

....

❀ **Sleep.** Did you get a decent night's sleep?

....

....

demands

✿ **Exercise.** Did you move your body today?

....

....

✿ **Routine.** Are you in a routine? Are you too bound to your routine?

....

....

✿ **Social contact.** Have you spoken to any friends or met up with anyone face to face today?

....

....

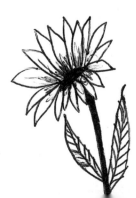

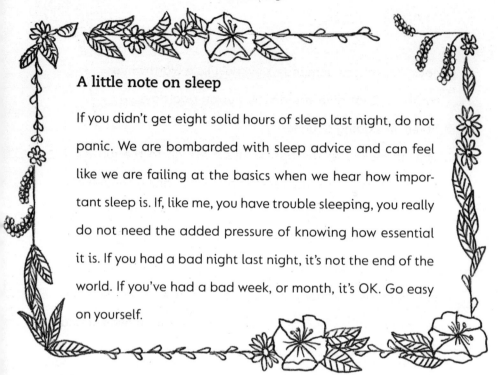

A little note on sleep

If you didn't get eight solid hours of sleep last night, do not panic. We are bombarded with sleep advice and can feel like we are failing at the basics when we hear how important sleep is. If, like me, you have trouble sleeping, you really do not need the added pressure of knowing how essential it is. If you had a bad night last night, it's not the end of the world. If you've had a bad week, or month, it's OK. Go easy on yourself.

Work, work, work

If you have a job, there is a strong possibility you will often feel stressed due to the demands that come with the territory. The stress might come from the amount you have to do in a day, the demands of your boss or colleagues, the expectations of the company or place of work, the people you have to direct and manage or work with, or simply not enjoying what the demands involve.

Whether you work as a team, are self-employed, are a civil servant or a volunteer, there will be demands that need to be met.

On good days those demands may feel like a worthwhile responsibility that give you a kick, but on bad days you might feel like doing a runner.

Having looked at the basics, let's move on to the job itself. Are the demands and subsequent stress outweighing the feelings of achievement, opportunities to learn, enjoyment, and sense of purpose? You might be nodding profusely already. Maybe you're not sure but know that something isn't quite right. I have certainly been there. I spent over twenty years feeling edgy due to the demands of live TV and radio, which at times annihilated the enjoyment and sense of achievement. As I became more well known and my work was seen and heard by bigger audiences, the pressure at times felt insurmountable. Teamed with the very low tolerance everyone seems to have for mistakes these days, I felt like I was in a straitjacket, and on constant high alert in case I said something wrong. The problem with having a job in the public eye is that you don't deal with your own feelings towards failure or a mistake in solitude: you do it alongside many others with firm opinions. All the enjoyment I had felt as a teenager, in my dream job, was drenched in anxiety.

Due to this pressure and stress my mental health took a battering in my early thirties, and I knew I needed to do something different. I believe cool people call this a 'pivot'. However you refer to it, I knew it was needed. It was not an easy decision, as I had a family to look after and no backup plan whatsoever, yet I knew I couldn't carry on as I had been. Jumping into the void felt scary and I definitely lost my confidence in those early days, but incrementally I have been able to build myself back up again, and through that process I have learned so much. It has taken me six years to build Happy Place from scratch and I still feel very much on the first rung of the ladder in terms of where I would like to take it. Personally, I believe it is never too late to pivot. Through my *Happy Place* podcast I have met so many people who have started over and dropped jobs that made them depressed or caused them mental and physical stress for something that felt better.

Recently Sir Bradley Wiggins came on to the *Happy Place* podcast and talked about retiring from cycling, as the pressure and press intrusion had made him very unhappy. Most would assume that when you're world class at something you would carry on for as long as possible, but when stress becomes unmanageable you often have no other choice but to try something different. I always love to use the example of my great friend Justine Jenkins, otherwise known as JJ, who worked in the city for years. She was making good money and had a high-flying social life, yet the stress began to take over. The high-octane nature of the job started to take its toll and she knew she needed to make changes. She had always been interested in make-up, so alongside her job in the city she started working for free doing make-up in theatres. This led to work on film sets, helping her collect great contacts in the world of make-up. After a lot of hard work, Justine is now one of the UK's most successful and in-demand make-up artists, and continues to campaign for the make-up industry to be animal cruelty-free and sustainable.

There seems to have been a recent influx of midlifers switching things up to gain more mental peace and motivation. Perhaps as the discussion around mental wellbeing increases more and more people are willing to make the leap. Yes, there is risk involved, yes there will be hard work and moments of feeling humbled from starting over again, but surely it's better than feeling trapped and miserable every day and burdened by the stressful demands of a job you hate? If you feel like your job isn't quite right for you, first up, you're not alone. Secondly, there is always room for movement, if only initially in tiny increments.

Through experiencing such a great change in my career, I have learned that it isn't about ridding yourself of all demands:

if anything, I have ended up with more when running my own brand. It's more about feeling the demands are worth it. The demands I face today feel worthwhile, as I feel challenged daily and can hopefully help others a bit too. My ideas of success have also greatly changed. Rather than attempting to quantify my achievements from how many people are watching me on TV or how perfect my performance is, I now gain an understanding of how things are going from the conversations I have with you lot. Every time I hear that my podcast or one of my books has helped somebody through a difficult patch, I feel motivated. It's a privilege I will never take for granted.

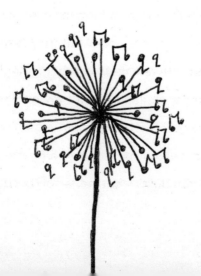

Interview with Nicole Crentsil

Meet Nicole Crentsil, founder of the UK's first festival to celebrate Black women, girls and non-binary people, Black Girl Fest. We were introduced a couple of years ago and have bonded over our work and aims for the future. Many, like myself, look up to Nicole and what she has achieved, but did her achievements come with a cost? How big is the stress and how does she keep on top of the demands?

Nicole, tell us a bit about your business and how you started it.

NC: I'm a Ghanaian-born British Black woman and I would say everything about who I am stems from my experience of navigating a world where I never really felt truly seen or heard. Growing up being 'different' led to me being singled out, which drew even more challenges with my own self-esteem and how I understood friendships, but mostly with who I wanted to be. I spent a large part of my younger years trying to fit into a world that didn't want me, simply because

I was Black. Assimilating into new cultures, languages and people made it hard for me to accept who I was or even who I could become, especially when everything around me did that for me already.

I guess that's why I feel so passionate about the work I do. For me, searching for community wasn't just for fun, but for necessity. Finding other Black women who have also been singled out or made to feel like their difference was a problem was actually my saving grace. Creating a business that actively works to make real change is my core mission. Black Girl Fest, which started as a huge annual celebration for Black women, has evolved into a brilliant creative studio, designing solutions that make Black women's lives better socially, economically and across educational spaces. I'm really proud of the projects we've rolled out and even prouder of the legacy we are leaving, not just for us, but for the future us.

As Black Girl Fest has grown, have you felt the stress grow with it?

Absolutely. I'm quite fearful of it, actually. In the business world everyone seems to have big ambitions to grow their business to have multiple global offices, with hundreds of teams and millions invested, and I honestly couldn't think of anything worse. I want my business to be small but mighty; compact but impactful.

The moment I decided this, most of my stress and the pressure this caused melted away. I quickly realised that one of the biggest stresses in running any business is expectation, either placed by society or ourselves. The media tells us what a 'good' CEO should look like, how they should speak, or what type of leader they should be. When really, we should be shaping ourselves based on what we want for ourselves. For me, I want to grow the business by our reach, impact and projects: this is my measurement of success.

How do you deal with the demands of organising such a big event?

Lots of sleep! For me, rest is really important, and when you're steering the ship it's really easy to keep working past

10pm. I also have a habit of doing things myself when I don't think tasks are done to a high standard, so learning to step away is really important. Finally, delegation! A really big one for me, especially as someone who likes to do everything. Delegating responsibilities is really key to managing my time, but also for prioritising that much-needed rest.

How do you cope with the needs of those around you and those who will be turning up to your events?

For me, it's really important that at all times we are mindful of individuals' specific needs, whether it may be access needs in or out of our spaces, parental support or if anyone should have an impairment preventing them from enjoying the event. Other than ensuring we have all bases covered, I'm also pretty big on boundaries. In the past I'd speak to everyone, give them all my attention, and then I'd feel emotionally burned out for weeks. I've realised that I can't be everything to everyone. I have to keep my space and do as little as I can but still seem approachable and friendly. I think having deep chats with everyone is not the one.

Does it ever feel lonely at the top? Some would assume that business owners and founders are less stressed than those employed, but you're responsible for other team members and a lot of communication with those you work with.

Oh, very, especially when you're doing it solo with no co-founder. The best way to combat this is having lots of other solo founder friends who you can lean on for advice, support or just to have a quick moan with. Having a mentor, adviser or role model also helps, especially if at times you don't feel centred in your path.

Having a break in responsibility is really key for me. Being the boss, making all the decisions and carrying the load of the mistakes is only for my work life and never for my home life. At home with my fiancé I specifically ask to not be making all the big decisions, to be waited on a little bit. I sort of get like a big kid, where I want to be taken care of, and it actually really works. I don't like being a boss babe or an independent woman at home; I think I would combust if I ever did.

When you are stressed, what helps?

Dancing! And lots of it. I really wish it was something more chilled like breathing work or yoga, but honestly playing really loud eighties power ballads and singing like the neighbours can't hear me is my fave thing to do. When that doesn't work, I pack things up and go to bed. There's nothing like pretending to quit and watching Netflix all day, knowing full well the work stress will be there when I return. For me, I get really overwhelmed when I take on too much, which leads to stress, so I try to say 'no' a lot more to help reduce this.

Is it possible to switch off, or do you find yourself thinking about work once you're home?

I think the working from home culture has made it a little harder to switch work off. It's a mixture for me: sometimes I work from home and get the most done because there are few distractions from my team. Other times, I get super lazy and end up not doing anything at all. It's a real balance and having some days in the office and some at home means each week is never the same. I've also stopped punishing myself for the days I work from home and get nothing done. If I'm resting and stationary while recharging my social battery, that seems like a whole lot of things I've got done.

Nicole makes a great point about rest and the guilt we can feel when we choose it over work. Rest is not culturally celebrated or seen as a productive endeavour, yet it can save the day when we are overwhelmed. Like Nicole, I can be tempted to push myself even when I know I'm close to burnout, but is it conducive to getting more done? I think not. Often when we reach the point of exhaustion, we end up setting ourselves back if we push through. We will cover the notion of rest more thoroughly later.

EVERYDAY DEMANDS

We know the big demands in life affect our stress levels hugely, but the small, incremental demands that chip away at our happiness and general wellbeing have a significant impact too. Getting stuck in traffic on the way to work is enough to make my blood boil on days when I am overtired. Having to organise a bunch of paperwork and pay parking fines or invoices can give me a headache if I already feel I'm behind on life admin.

I think speed has a lot to do with how we handle the everyday demands of life. If you haven't read the beautiful book *The Things You Can See Only When You Slow Down* by Haemin Sunim, it's a gorgeous and essential read. We might not feel we have the option to change the speed at which we move when we are running late, or have too much to do, but is there more potential to slow down than we believe? Sometimes I want to race through the day so I can get to the bit where I sit on the sofa numbing myself with TV. I feel a sense of safety wrapped up in the drama of someone else's life on a reality show, comforted by a cocoon of blissful ignorance about my own stress. I am, in fact, no safer in these moments than I was during a busier part of the day. Slow down and don't race to the end of the day, then see what you notice and how the speed at which you move affects your reaction to stressful situations.

Little things to slow down your pace

❀ **Eat without distractions.** Don't watch the TV or flick through emails on your phone. Enjoy each flavour and texture and take your time. I just did this very thing with a slice of peanut butter on toast. Delish.

❀ **Breathe with intention every few minutes.** Take a long, deep breath in and out. If you do this throughout your day you will catch yourself in moments of rushing where you may be holding your breath.

❀ **Bring your senses to the party.** When we rush, we miss everything going on around us. Throughout the day, take short moments to notice the colours around you: the smells, the sounds, and how your body feels within your clothes, or how the air feels on your skin. Jot down what you noticed about your day. What did you smell? What colours jumped out at you? What sounds felt challenging and which ones felt blissful?

Breathe easy

Let's look at everyday demands that don't seem like a huge deal in the moment, but build up incrementally over time. Your email inbox may be bulging or the washing basket full to the brim; you may have several phone calls to make that you're not looking forward to; or maybe you cannot get your children to go to sleep at night. Each one of these small pressures can easily lead to overwhelm and big stress. In these everyday moments of stress, we can help ourselves by doing one very simple thing: we can breathe. For those of you that have not tried breathwork, it may sound overly simple and obvious. But in these moments of stress, we so often forget to breathe. Instead, we tense up our muscles, screw up our foreheads, and hold our breath at the top or bottom of an inhale or exhale. Reducing the amount of oxygen we take in causes our physical bodies even more stress, so the whole scenario becomes a cyclical vortex of tension. Many of you may have already tried breathwork practices but might need a nudge to weave the concept throughout your everyday.

I remember once visiting a therapist at a time in my life where I was experiencing panic attacks very frequently. I felt on edge a lot of the time and stressful situations made me feel like I was leaving my own body. The therapist met me in the reception of his office, then we took a short walk out of the door, up a flight of stairs to his treatment room. As I sat down, his first words were: 'You haven't taken a breath since I shook your hand in reception.' I had gotten very used to subconsciously holding my breath when I was nervous, as if it might freeze time and save me from my own fate. Breathing at times felt like a luxury I didn't have. There wasn't the time or space for it.

The therapist's observation acted as a wake-up call. I started to track how often I held my breath and what the triggers of stress were each time. When I noticed it, I could make the active decision to breathe deeply. I would then feel my shoulders drop with the breath, my eyes soften slightly and the tension in my bones dissipate. The next time you are late or can't find a parking spot or are on a packed train, notice how you are breathing. Are your breaths shallow and quick, or are you holding your breath at the top of an inhale?

MY BREATHING IS ...

Little things to help calm the nervous system

I am very fortunate that in my recent line of work I have met many breathwork experts who have helped me understand the power of breath and how it can help us to work through stress, anger, sorrow and more. Rebecca Dennis has studied breathwork for many years and has created some beautiful therapeutic sessions for you on the Happy Place app. They are only short, maybe ten minutes in length, but you would be surprised how impactful even short sessions are when it comes to stress reduction.

Give it a go now. Rebecca often advises people to use 'box breathing' to calm the physical body and mind: take a breath in for four, and then hold your breath for four at the top of your inhale. Breathe out again for four, and then hold your breath for four at the bottom of your exhale. Do this for as long as you feel necessary and notice how you feel.

Are your thoughts moving at a slower pace? Does your body feel calmer and less tense?

THERE'S NO ROOM

Many studies tell us that social interaction is one of the foundations of good general wellbeing. It can help with a feeling of connection, with our levels of happiness, stress reduction and more. *The Good Life* by Marc Schulz and Robert J. Waldinger is an amazing book about human connection and relationships, if you want to read more on this subject. It's based on the longest study carried out on human happiness and reveals that solid relationships not only boost us mentally but affect our physical health too. Knowing how important decent relationships are, you may assume we all need a large circle of friends and a buzzing social life. But balance is key. What if you already feel overloaded with interaction? What if you actually just need some alone time?

My house is a constant hive of activity. My *Happy Place* podcast is recorded here with my brilliant team and different guests each week, with my kids bursting through the door after school, Jesse running his business from our home, builders everywhere and the doorbell constantly ringing. You get the picture. I adore meeting new people and having a buzz in the home but sometimes I crave solitude. I'm sure many of you can relate to feeling like there isn't quite enough space for you to properly digest the day, unwind or simply sit and be. When I've had a very busy time at work, alongside juggling school life and excessive amounts of kids' parties at weekends, I can feel myself reaching boiling point. My stress levels rise like a stormy sea, and I know it's time for me to make some space.

If I'm really short on time, just a half-hour walk in the park alone gives me a little space. If I have longer, I will read on my own for hours, listen to music (going through a heavy Shania Twain phase right now) and walk miles. When my kids are older, maybe I'll have time to go to the coast on my own or take a short overnight break. That doesn't feel possible at the moment, so mini-breaks in the day feel important to allow me solitude in busy times.

How much time do you spend on your own each week and how does it make you feel?

....

....

....

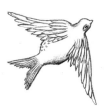

Little things to help create space

❋ **Carve out some daily alone time.** Most days I set an alarm for 6am, knowing that on a school day I don't have to wake the kids until 6:30. This gives me a full 30 minutes of screen-free alone time (bar Simon the cat). I make a coffee, feed Simon, and listen to the birds outside. It's usually the only portion of the day when I am not needed by anyone, uncontactable and free to do as I please. That 30 minutes gives me space and time to get in the right frame of mind for the rest of my day. Where do you think you could find small pockets of space in your day or week? Could you fit in a lunchtime walk? Or a ten-minute meditation before bed?

❋ **Give yourself a break.** I don't smoke and, although I would never advocate for anyone to take it up, I often feel envious of the small break created by the habit. When I'm working from home and don't have time for a walk I take fag-free fag breaks. I step outside of my tiny studio, which is airless and sometimes stuffy, and take deep breaths outside for a couple of minutes to reset my mind and stretch my legs. It's incredible what even a short break in the fresh air can do for our stress levels.

❋ **Don't feel scared to ask for time alone if you feel you need it.** It's become something of a modern-day myth that you have to spend every waking hour with your partner. If you are married or in a relationship and feel you need space, do not hesitate to ask for it. Go on a date night on your own, take a solo walk to clear your head, or watch a film in bed in solitude. There is no shame in it and if you explain to your partner that you need space to regain energy and have a proper rest, they shouldn't take it personally. In her book, *The Book of Boundaries*, Melissa Urban, who I mentioned earlier, gives many examples of how setting boundaries with other people helps our stress levels. If we are constantly people-pleasing and saying yes to the demands of others, we will end up feeling more stressed, full of resentment and strung out. Telling others what you need and saying no when you need to claw back space and time is essential.

When Kate Ferdinand was a guest on the *Happy Place* podcast recently, we talked about ways to navigate overwhelm as a parent, but I think her advice stands up in any situation where you are craving space. She said that for her to parent well, she has to have time away from the kids. She finds it hard to believe she deserves it and sometimes feels guilty, yet she knows it's essential so she can give her five children the love and attention they need. You may not have children or stepchildren yourself; perhaps you live with your partner or flatmate. You may find things even more complicated if you work from home too. Whatever your set-up, if you need space then ask for it. If you feel nervous about asking for space, that's OK. It might be a new concept for you. Honesty is always best, so approach your partner/flatmate/relative and explain where your head is at, and that you feel you need time in solitude to process, reflect and gain some mental peace. No one can argue with that.

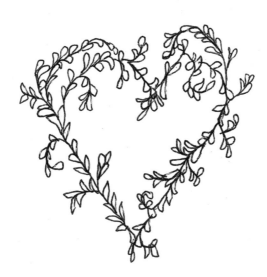

LIFE ADMIN

When speaking to an incredibly good friend about this book, we set about comparing the parts of life we find the most stressful. He is a freelance writer, director and actor who moves about a lot. The demands change daily, but one that causes constant stress for him is life admin and paperwork. He described the feeling of having a pile of paperwork to sort through as if he were drowning in it all. If this resonates, you may find your coping mechanism is to leave it all in a pile, unread and un-dealt with. Which life admin jobs are you putting off? Make a list below, prioritising the order of what needs to be done first.

1 ....

2 ....

3 ....

4 ....

5 ....

6 ....

7 ....

8 ....

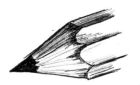

Little things to help deal with life admin

If tackling this list feels insurmountable, you could rope in a friend. Why not task them with the same job, and text or call them afterwards so you can congratulate each other?

Sometimes I will offer myself a small treat to inspire me to get the job done, like you would an unruly dog. If I know I have a ton of emails to do and invoices to sort out, yet can feel myself moving towards procrastination, I will imagine a hot chocolate afterwards or an episode of *Motherland* awaiting me on the sofa. Set yourself manageable goals each day to chip away at any life admin and reward yourself for the effort applied. It's win-win. Life admin sorted, less stress and a treat! Woof.

Jot down how you imagine you will feel once it is all done. When those letters or bills have been sorted, parking fines paid, emails replied to or doctors' appointments finally booked, how will you feel then?

....

....

....

HEALTH

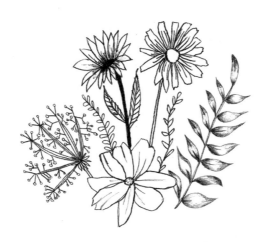

Stress is not only an undesirable emotional response because it feels uncomfortable in the moment, it also affects our physical and mental health if not dealt with. Watching a recent episode of Rich Roll's podcast on YouTube, with guest Dr Rangan Chatterjee, I learned that anywhere between 70 and 90 per cent of all conditions seen by a primary care doctor on any given day are caused by stress. That seems like a big percentage and something we need to address to give ourselves a better chance of good health, both physical and mental. These conditions could range from depression and anxiety to low libido, inflammation issues, insomnia, hormonal problems, diabetes and more. There can be other factors at play but Dr Chatterjee insists that stress usually has a part in it all.

It can be a terrifying thought, but when we recognise the long-term effects of stress, it can also be empowering. Rather than feeling floored by worry about how stress might manifest itself in mental or physical issues, we can think back to what Dr Jud explained earlier and begin to cultivate awareness as to how we respond to the stressful situations in our life. Often, we cannot change a stressful situation, rid ourselves of stressful people or move from a stressful job right away, but we do have the power to change how we respond to it. If we also think back to Owen's advice, positive self-talk is imperative when it comes to moving through stressful situations. So let's keep that in mind as we look more closely at the mind/body connection.

It used to be seen as a little far out to assume mental or emotional stress could manifest physically, yet these days there is so much data and science to prove that stress can evolve into ill health. You might be able to track obvious outcomes of stress in your physical body already. At any given time, I only have to peer down at my own hands to calibrate how stressed I am. The skin around my fingers will be red and broken when I'm full of nerves and running on adrenaline. It's almost an involuntary response to my emotional stress when I pick the skin and dig at the painful rawness beneath. I can also sense my chest tightening and feel small pinpricks on my scalp. If things are bad, the stress shows up as headaches, constipation, insomnia, colds and mouth ulcers. These are all warning signs that I need to calm my nervous system and potentially make some changes.

Stress can also manifest in mental health issues, such as OCD, anxiety and depression. I went through a stressful situation over ten years ago that resulted in a period of depression and intrusive thoughts I seemingly had no control over. Although I have moved through that acute period of stress, there's still an anxiety that lingers. For a long time I was unsure as to why I was having panic attacks, but recently I received an OCD diagnosis, which has been a bit of a revelation. Without getting too tied up in the label, I am now able to see how my brain works more clearly. When I am having extremely worrying thoughts, which often lead to panic, I try to reach for 'oh this is OCD, it's not a real threat or concern'. Sometimes that shortens the period of panic, but it's still early days, so often I cannot override the compulsion to check a lock on a window, or the gas rings on the oven. Once again, I'm a work in progress. Somewhere down the line, during stressful periods, my brain has learned to worry big. It's something I'm still attempting to understand better and rectify where I can, with self-compassion.

The flavour of stress we need to keep a check on is long-term stress – the kind that's buried in our bones. It's the stress you become so used to that you don't remember life without it. This takes its toll on the physical body and affects our mental health, and it needs to be addressed when we feel we can do so. It's not easy to unpick years of built-up stress, nor is it quick to change ingrained habits, but it is doable with a little help and support and, of course, desire. I have to remind myself of this all the time. I force-feed myself the words *I have a choice* to remind myself that some of my reactions are habitual. If you're willing to try to change inbuilt habits to address long-term stress, in order to keep physically and mentally well, so am I. In this chapter, let's take a deeper dive into habits and the little things we can do to help ourselves stay healthy.

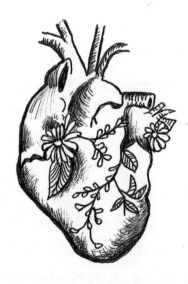

WARNING SIGNAL

If you feel scared or freaked out knowing how much stress can impact the mind and physical body, that's normal. What we don't need here is more for you to worry about, so let's reframe this realisation and see the physical reactions to stress as warning signs. We can all habitually fall into cycles of stress, sometimes so much so that we don't even realise how much pressure we are under. We plough through the day in fight or flight mode, thinking it's totally normal. Luckily the body is there to tell us things are not OK and that a recalibration is needed. The book *The Body Keeps the Score* dives into this subject in great depth, with author Bessel van der Kolk explaining how those who have suffered trauma in life can often find their bodies stuck in fight or flight mode. His therapies and methods help those who are in mental and physical stress to feel a sense of freedom in their minds and bodies.

Your own warning signs may show up so often that you're used to them or ignore them altogether. In this section of the book, we will try to identify the physical issues you might experience, but also look at the little things you can do to lessen the stress you are feeling. Your stress might show up as physical fatigue, joint problems, gut issues, inflammation, skin issues, back pain, and so on.

Can you detect how stress might show up physically for you? If so, write a little about this below.

....

....

....

....

....

....

....

....

....

TAKING ITS TOLL

What we don't need is even more pressure to NOT FEEL STRESSED. I don't want this section of the book to make any of us feel more desperate about lowering our stress levels. Instead, this part will hopefully act as a guide to how we can spot stress in the body and what coping mechanisms can help us take back control in order to feel more physically in balance.

The work of Dr Joe Dispenza has been transformative for those seeking help and healing as well as those wanting to prevent stress manifesting in a physical sense. His own story of physical healing runs parallel with the anecdotes of others he shares, and illustrates the importance of understanding the connection between the mind and body. During a triathlon Joe was seriously injured when a car hit him from behind and broke six of his vertebrae. This traumatic moment led to Joe's exploration of the world of mental strength, healing and meditation. Now physically back to full health, he helps others heal from past pain, cope with current stresses and cultivate a mindset that allows optimum health. If you are interested to learn more, Joe has many interesting YouTube videos and books on his teachings, featuring anecdotes of those he has helped.

Before I had any self-awareness and knowledge on this topic, I used to end up in a state of physical imbalance constantly. In my mid-twenties, amidst a relentless seven-day working week with very little rest, commentary from the press and not enough self-care, all leading to a lack of self-esteem, my stress levels were high. My life from the outside looked pretty good, with an exciting job, a little cottage for me and my cats to safely live in and food in the fridge. Yet my response to the environment I was working in was one of heightened stress. I recall being on a photoshoot, sitting in the make-up chair, staring at myself blankly in the mirror. It was as if my whole body was rigid and frozen, my vital organs in catatonic tension. I was constipated and I had cystitis.

Let's not beat around the bush here: when you cannot go to the toilet in either manner, it is pretty miserable. You may be reading this with a large sigh of relief if you've had or currently have a similar lack of movement internally. Thankfully, I was able to very slowly make changes to the areas of life that were causing me great stress. I moved out of workplaces that filled me with terror. I stopped saying yes to everything out of fear I would never work again, and no to things that made me feel horrid.

Little things to help you answer from a place that feels right to you

❋ **Say yes to things that mentally and physically make you feel lighter and open.** Remember what Dr Jud said at the start of the book about openness.

❋ **Remember that those around you don't have to understand or agree with your decisions;** it's most important that those decisions feel right *to you*.

❋ **Know that you deserve to say no to things you don't want and yes to things you really do.**

Making a decision that is right for you might lead to an awkward conversation, telling someone no, or walking down an unknown path. My friend, the author and wellness expert Donna Lancaster, calls those uncomfortable moments *bum clenchers*. Feeling uncomfortable shouldn't be enough to stop you making that decision. Usually, initial discomfort makes way for long-term peace, knowing you've made the decision for all the right reasons.

Is there a risk you need to take to live authentically? Do you need to say no to someone, or something? Or yes to a new path?

On a scale of 1–10, how uncomfortable does actioning your decision make you feel?

....

Do you think it's worth moving through the discomfort? If so, why?

....

....

If your answer to that last question is yes, GO DO IT. Make that change, know that it might be uncomfortable along the way, but also that it will help reduce your long-term stress levels. If you have decided to make a change, no matter how small, come back in a few weeks or months to this section of the book and compare your physical symptoms of stress then to how they are today. Write down what you notice.

....

....

....

Interview with my mum, Lin

My mum knows only too well how mental stress can impact the body, as she was diagnosed with polymyalgia six years ago. This condition causes extreme pain, stiffness and inflammation in the muscles and joints. Inflammation is one of the most common physical outcomes of stress and Mum's diagnosis related directly to her joints. She has endured a lot of pain, hospital appointments and medication, but is now in a much better place mentally and physically. Meet Lin.

Mum, I'm keen to learn more about your polymyalgia and what you have learned from it. What symptoms were you experiencing before your diagnosis?

LC: It started with the odd twinge in the back. During a yoga session I realised that when I lay on the floor it hurt, and it quickly progressed to pain all over the body. I thought it may be something a chiropractor could help with, but no, it wasn't. I then went to the doctor, who sent me for a blood test. All this time the pain was getting worse and worse all over my body, accompanied by stiffness where I couldn't even move my neck from side to side. I needed help getting out of bed, dressing, climbing the stairs and getting out of the car. I felt ancient.

How did the pain affect your mental health and stress levels?

Experiencing pain this severe and for so long – five years – led to even more depression. I managed to get an appointment with a rheumatologist, who diagnosed polymyalgia and said that on average it lasts approximately two years and then burns itself out. Before its natural burnout I was to take steroids every day on a reducing dose. The steroids helped with the pain, but as soon as I reduced them the inflammation would flare up again, so I went back to the original dosage. It was all a bit of a balancing act.

How did you begin to recover?

After around five years, when I was on a very low dose of steroids, I could feel I was turning a corner, and then one day I felt fine. It had, luckily, burned itself out.

How much of your diagnosis do you believe was caused by emotional stress?

I 100 per cent believe stress caused my physical illness. That understanding has helped me heal and make changes. I am no longer on medication for this condition, but I think it would have been impossible to manage the pain without it. I feel great, in fact I feel better now than when I did before all this happened to me.

I believe stress played a huge part in why I developed polymyalgia: the constant anxiety started to impact me on a very physical level, and more than likely took my immune system down. I don't think I dealt with the stress in my life over the years. I knew it was there but I ignored it to a degree, hence the physical attack on my body.

We now have a completely different lifestyle: we are almost stress-free apart from the stuff that every human being experiences. We eat well, walk for miles in the amazing surroundings we live in, we have a gorgeous rescue dog, we surround ourselves with good people and appreciate everything we have. Life is very good.

I am so glad and grateful that my mum is doing well and not in so much physical pain anymore. I know it's taken a lot of work for Mum to make certain changes and manage her stress levels and it's still something she has to keep in check today. I hope hearing Mum talk openly about her physical challenges and improvements gives you hope that it's sometimes possible to improve your physical health by making positive changes.

As Mum mentioned, she and my dad walk for miles each day, which is hugely beneficial to them. If you want to read about the most incredible story of physical healing, I urge you to read Raynor Winn's book *The Salt Path*, which charts not only Raynor's recovery from homelessness but also how walking for miles every day helped her husband Moth's chronic physical illness. Raynor also appeared on my *Happy Place* podcast as a guest, to retell this beautiful story that will stay with me forever.

Mum and Dad also have the love and companionship of their rescue dog, Wilma. Animals have long been a transformative tonic to humans and can help reduce stress greatly. I have experienced this time and time again with my own cats. Simon, who heavily features on my Instagram, is our rescue cat and has brought the whole family so much love, joy and calm. Most animals are masters at soothing.

TRAUMA

At the start of the health section, I mentioned long-term stress and how it can impact our physical bodies. Mum's story also backs up how years of unprocessed pain can manifest physically.

Sometimes that long-term stress is caused by trauma. Healing from earth-shattering events is a much more complex and longer endeavour, yet it is possible. I have been fortunate enough to speak with so many individuals who have overcome traumatic events. This isn't to say they live without any hangovers from the past. I think what I've learned is that you find coping mechanisms to deal with the aftershock.

During a challenging time in my early thirties, I started to react to stress very physically. Because I wasn't processing the challenges I faced, I began experiencing panic attacks and insomnia. Sleep still often evades me, so I create many conditions to help me cope, but they usually only worsen the problem. To unpick it all means to see the fear beneath it. Although sleep is unrelated to the previous challenges I faced, it represents a residue of fear. This is why I believe that in order to lessen my sleep issues I need to focus on feeling safe in all areas. The safer I feel the less stressed I will feel.

Little things that can help you feel safe

✽ **Talk to someone.** Tell them how you are feeling physically and mentally. Talk through the times when you feel unsafe or scared.

✽ **Go easy on yourself.** What we don't need in these moments is to berate ourselves for not coping. Let's remind ourselves of the importance of positive self-talk that Owen mentioned at the start of the book. Your fear in these moments is valid, so go easy on yourself.

✽ **Know you're not alone.** When I'm experiencing insomnia in the middle of the night, I try to think about all of those people who are working night shifts. I feel a sense of camaraderie with their sleeplessness and tiredness. I think about all the parents up with awake children or babies. I am much kinder to myself in these moments because I don't feel so alone with it all.

✽ **EMDR (Eye Movement Desensitisation and Reprocessing).** This form of therapy has helped me reduce my stress and anxiety, but I still have work to do. It's an incredibly powerful therapy where side to side eye movements or bilateral tapping help recalibrate the mind and lessen the sting of painful memories.

If you are dealing with trauma from the past, do not feel beaten when you can't control the physical symptoms of the stress caused. That will only leave you feeling defeated and potentially more stressed. Healing from trauma or very challenging experiences takes time, support and acceptance. The acceptance part might be the hardest cog in the process. I find it hard to accept that I can't always control the physical manifestation of stress at night. I also find it difficult to remain patient in the process of healing. This is all entirely normal. Go easy on yourself; know it might take time and that the speed of your recovery is irrelevant.

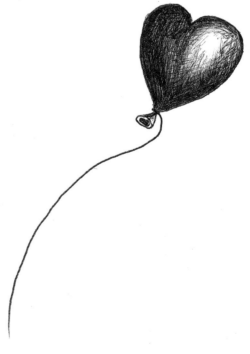

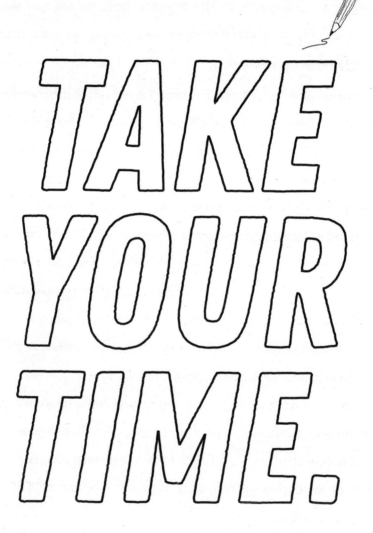

SLEEP

A little note on insomnia

There is no amount of lavender spray, herbal tea or otherwise that will touch the sides when you have sleep issues. I have slathered myself in magnesium and chugged cherry tonic. It goes deeper than that. Many sleep issues derive from stress or are purely psychological. It will never do any harm to relax the body to aid your sleep, but a full mind/body approach is often needed. There is one technique that focuses more on the psychological side and it is a tip I learned from Deepak Chopra on the *Happy Place* podcast. I essentially used this episode as a private therapy session with the great Chopra and quizzed him on my night-time panic. His advice was to stop resisting the fear and panic. To welcome it in. It wasn't the answer I was anticipating but it really does help; as soon as you stop fighting the panic, it slightly subsides. It might not go entirely but it is a much more peaceful route than berating yourself for the panic or increasing the fear of it. Whatever you resist, PERSISTS. Thank you, Deepak.

Another little note on sleep, actually

Watch how much stress you are willingly taking on before bed. Are you watching stressful, violent, or edgy TV shows in bed? Are you reading distressing literature? Are you on your phone moments before you go to sleep?

Because I have historically had trouble sleeping, I am a total bore before bed. Get ready to read about the most rigid and dull bedtime routine ever.

- 9pm, turn phone off. That's right, it goes OFF.
- Take two magnesium tablets.
- Read in bed for 30 minutes. Gentle, lovely books only.
- Go for a wee. Maybe twice, just in case.
- Pop in earplugs.
- Eye mask on.
- Lights out by 10pm.

God, I'm bored just typing that out. Maybe you've fallen asleep reading the list; that would be a bit of a bonus! Yet I know that for me to have a stress-free night, the run-up to bedtime has to be as consistent as possible. What would you like your night-time routine to look like?

MY NIGHTTIME ROUTINE

Little things to help with sleep

* **Cut out blue light.** I know that if I allow tons of blue light from my phone or laptop before bed, I will not sleep. If you like to watch TV or a laptop at night you can buy glasses that cut out the blue light emitted from your screen. You may find these helpful.

* **Avoid sugar close to bedtime.** I'm also careful not to eat anything too sugary before bed as it will lead to a spike in energy, which I really do not need.

* **Be mindful of what you watch.** Check that the media you're watching before bed isn't too distressing or stimulating.

Those of you who work nights, irregular hours or have small kids, I HEAR YOU. I often have to work at night if I'm hosting an event or doing a podcast with someone in another time zone. I also have a son with similar sleep issues to me, so a full night's sleep is almost unheard of in our house. So I aim for consistency where I can. It doesn't have to be perfect, so I try not to feel worried if on some nights my routine is broken. I've also learned through experience that you can have a jolly good day on very little sleep. Sometimes I write off a whole day if I've not slept well. In a dramatic cry I will lament that there is no point even trying to achieve happiness on such a day but go on to experience quite the opposite.

It's also interesting that what we do in the day massively impacts how we sleep. Recently I interviewed sleep expert Dr Sophie Bostock, who has created many tips and sessions for sleeping on our Happy Place app. She explained that one of the best things we can do for a good night's sleep is to expose ourselves to natural daylight first thing in the morning. It need only be for a few minutes, but even that short amount of time in natural light will help support our circadian rhythms. If you work at a desk, could you move it to face a window, so you have natural light pouring in to where you are seated? Can you decrease your caffeine intake in the day too? All of these little things will have a big impact on your sleep, which should make for less stress at night and also for the next day.

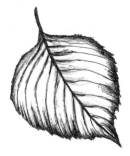

YOUR BODY

Let's get physical with a meditative body scan. Unlike a medical scan that allows us to *see* problematic areas, this introspective technique helps us to tune into where we *feel* tension in our bodies.

If you have worked your way through this chapter and still can't detect where the stress might live in your body, let's take things one step further. Are you the sort of person who lives more in your head than your body, or someone that feels a lot physically but might push certain thoughts aside? Some of us will ruminate obsessively, run over things from the past, churn over ideas, and get lost in memories or future fears. There's a lot of action in the brain and the rest of the body can get forgotten about.

This is 100 per cent how I work. When my mind is whirring non-stop, I become oblivious to how my body is reacting to my thoughts and where the stress is affecting me physically. As I know I have a propensity to live in my head, I try to cultivate times where I am less in the mind and more in the body. Welcome, the body scan. It doesn't take long and is always surprising.

Body Scan

If you can, lie down or sit in a comfy chair. Lying down is always preferable as you can really feel into your spine.

Start at the top of your head. In your mind, scan your head for any stress, pain or discomfort. Is there tension behind the eyes? Is your forehead all scrunched up? Notice how your jaw feels, too, as many of us carry tension in this area.

Now move to your neck and shoulders. I don't know about you, but my shoulder blades feel like metal rods today; heavy and uncomfortable. So much of my stress sits heavy on my shoulders.

Now move to your chest and take some deep breaths to examine how your lungs are feeling. Is there any tightness or restriction?

Move down the body to the gut, pelvis, thighs, calves and feet, scanning for tension and stress as you go. Don't hold any judgement if there is stress. Remember, you don't want this to cause more stress. If you do feel tension, you're not doing anything wrong or failing some kind of test. Just notice where it sits.

little things

On the picture of the body below, mark all the areas where you can feel tension and physical stress.

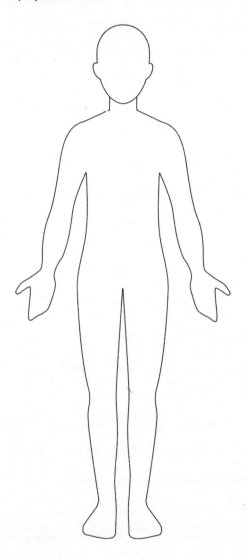

Next time you are dealing with a stressful situation, actively drop into your physical body. Focus your thoughts on that body part and breathe into it. Can you visualise breath moving down to that area of tension? Visualisation is a powerful tool to use in these moments. Breathe into it and exhale the stress. Do this for as long as you need to.

What are you eating?

Nutrition is a huge subject and one I have deeply dived into for my own healing. If you have followed my work over the years, you may have heard me talking about the ten-year period where I was bulimic. The illness itself showed up in varying degrees of severity over that decade, with a ferocious start to the problem surfacing at the age of 19 and a more sporadic experience later in my twenties. It was undoubtedly born out of stress, as I navigated a period of life where I felt entirely out of control. My work life was a rush of high expectations and attention and my personal life full of chaotic relationships. The bulimia felt like a release from it all. A way out of the chaos. A secret no one else had access to.

It sadly wasn't a way out of the chaos and after a few years that I spent in a trance, believing it was my only way to cope, I started to feel the internal stress it was causing. External stress may have ignited the problem but the action itself was causing my body stress that really started to show. Our body tends to shout about stuff when it needs attention and mine was doing that a lot during this period. I had gum issues (which I still must be mindful of today), and my digestion was understandably out of sync. The stress my body was under was not sustainable, so at the age of 29 I began a long road to recovery.

Being a very all-or-nothing person, I pored over cookbooks and learned as much as I could about nutrition to help with my fear of certain foods. I cooked, baked, chopped and blended every combination of scary food I could get my hands on. I wanted my body to heal and for the internal stress to dissipate. I'm still hugely motivated by this period of my life and am constantly wanting to learn about nutrition and how much of an impact it has on our bodies and mental health.

Food magic

The magical thing about food is that it doesn't just help maintain physical health or heal old wounds; it can also lower stress levels and improve our mental health. There is so much research these days about which foods can boost mood, help with concentration and lessen anxiety. The first step in understanding how our bodies react to food is to have an awareness of what we are eating. I do not align with diets that purport to give you a flat stomach or eliminate unwanted jowls. I'm interested in nutrition and what can support our physical and mental health in the best conceivable way. I have also found that cooking is a highly enjoyable activity that takes up all of my concentration and feels almost meditative. I love nothing more than to follow an intricate cake recipe methodically; my mind fixed on measurements and not on exterior stresses.

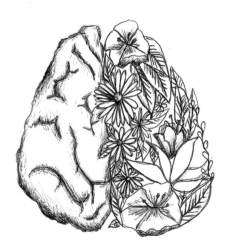

MY FOOD DIARY

Write down everything you have eaten today. Do this without judgement or worry – I'm certainly not judging you. Next to each meal or snack, jot down how it made you feel. Did it give you an energy boost, leave you feeling flat and low or make you tired?

Breakfast:

Lunch:

Dinner:

Snacks:

Drinks:

How foods can help reduce stress and anxiety

If you are looking to lower stress and anxiety, here are some foods that can help:

1 Leafy greens, as they are rich in magnesium.

2 Nuts and seeds and whole grains, as they are slow in releasing their energy.

3 Foods rich in zinc, such as cashews and egg yolk.

4 Sweet potatoes are nutrient-rich carbs that may help lower cortisol levels.

5 Fermented foods such as kimchi are packed with beneficial probiotics that interact with gut bacteria. Changes to gut microbes can directly affect mood.

6 Eggs are full of amino acids and vitamins that are needed for a healthy stress response.

7 Fatty fish, like mackerel and salmon, is full of omega-3s, which help your body and mind handle stress. Taking omega-3 supplements (or if you are vegan like me, the vegan alternative) is great for focus and clarity.

8 If you're vegan, swap fish and eggs out for chickpeas. They're bursting with vitamins and minerals, like magnesium and potassium, that can help with mental performance.

9 Herbal teas are great for relaxing before bed or in stressful times too. My favourite is ginger.

Check out Kimberley Wilson's incredible book *Unprocessed* for more information on how food affects our mood and mental health. It's an exceptional read.

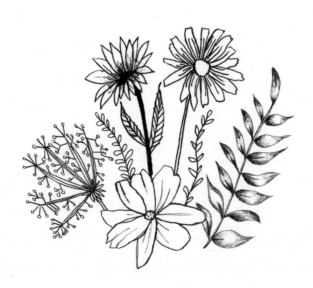

Little things to help you eat well

If you feel overwhelmed about changing how you eat, try some little things that feel easy but worthwhile:

❀ Freeze your favourite fruits and then in the morning chuck them in a blender with a spoonful of protein-rich almond butter and the milk of your choice. You can also add in some frozen spinach to up your leafy greens.

❀ One of my favourite easy meals is dahl. I bung red lentils, garlic, ginger, tinned tomatoes, curry powder, soy sauce and stock into a pan and let it all simmer for 15 minutes. It's quick, cheap and full of protein, fibre and flavour.

❀ Soups are always a good way to get a lot of colourful veg into your system and they're perfect for a cold day.

Here's the real kicker. When we are stressed mentally, we are much more likely to make bad choices in all areas of life – to pick up the biscuits, neck the wine, eat too quickly and so on. When I'm feeling stressed, I crave processed vegan cheese slices on the whitest, most processed bread, so white it looks fake, all washed down with the sweetest, most sugar-laden hot chocolate possible. When we are stressed, we want comfort, and that comfort normally comes from sugar and over-processed foods.

Of course, there is no harm in enjoying a vegan cheese slice sarnie every now and then, but if comfort eating becomes a habit we often lean on, we might find ourselves feeling physically worse than we did before. I used to comfort eat on TV sets when I was a teenager. I felt nervous and out of my depth and there were bags of sweets everywhere in the green room. I would uncon-sciously eat until I felt slightly nauseous from the sugar. I still find myself reaching for chocolate when I get stuck on a book edit and start feeling the stress creep in. Each delicious bite offers a sweet escape and a numbness that only delays dealing with the stress I'm feeling.

Most of us do it, but if you believe it is causing your physical body harm or is prompting more mental stress, then try pausing before you reach for the snack. Feel the stress, notice what is caus-ing it, then pause. You might notice that the compulsion dissipates naturally. Dr Jud talked about riding this wave at the start of the book. See if, after a minute or so, your compulsion lessens. You can do the same with cigarettes, alcohol or anything else you are using to lessen the feeling of stress.

Foods made with refined sugar, ones that are highly processed, like alcohol, are also all very addictive, so it's no wonder we turn to them when we feel stressed out and in need of comfort.

Little things that help change habits

❈ Remembering it's just a habit enables us to make more beneficial choices. In that pause, could you just simply feel your feelings? What's the worst that can happen? Notice the stress, the acerbic inner voice, the pain. Just let it be there. I remember reading a passage in Tara Brach's book *Trusting the Gold* on how to tell your negative thoughts and emotions that they belong. Trying to banish them causes resistance and tension, whereas just letting them be doesn't.

❈ Eat some fruit or have a big glass of water instead of going to comfort food. For those with eating problems I must state I am talking about avoiding comfort eating rather than essential meals and healthy snacks throughout the day. Sugary, processed foods usually make us feel worse and stress the gut out, which can lead to constipation or digestion issues and keep us in a loop of craving. Pick something you know will make you feel energised and boosted. This isn't about denying ourselves of all comfort and pleasure, it's about noticing when food is working for us and against us.

❀ Remember this is not about how much you eat, or about restricting yourself: it's about making choices that support your immune system, digestion, and all-round wellbeing so you feel less physically and mentally stressed. Then when you have a treat, like my beloved hot chocolate, you really enjoy it, rather than gulping it down to drown the stress.

❀ If you are currently living with an eating disorder, do seek professional help if you haven't already. I wish you well on your road to recovery.

MOVING YOUR BODY

I know it's obvious, but exercise helps with physical and mental stress. We all know this, but we might not actually do it. It doesn't matter what it is: we just need to move our bodies (if we can). Over the years my relationship with exercise has changed hugely. Previously I thought that unless I was panting and on my knees in a puddle of my own sweat, then it wasn't worth it. I couldn't be further from that mindset these days. I don't want to punish my body – I did enough of that back in the day – and I know that gentle and simple ways of moving are going to be just as beneficial.

My favourite method is simply walking. If I am at home writing, recording podcasts or editing I will always try, either in my lunch break or right at the start of the day, to get a walk in. I have never regretted a walk and always come home feeling better. I often use this time to reflect and work through my stresses too. Just today, on an early morning walk after the school run, I was processing a stress-ful situation involving a couple of people who I find challenging. I was having a fantasy argument with them in my head and running through what I might say if I bumped into them. This situation had been bubbling under the surface all week and I was starting to feel the physical stress manifest in low-level headaches and back pain. On this walk I breathed deeply, let my feet carry me across crunchy, icy ground and with each step felt a little less stressed. A walk gives us time and distance from a stressful situation which subsequently helps us to *respond rather than react to stress.*

Little things to help get you moving

To move your body, you do not need to join a gym, already have a high level of fitness, or push yourself too much. It can be small moments: a dance in the kitchen to your favourite music, a walk with a mate or a swim if you live by the sea. What do you like doing? Whatever it is, do more of that.

A note on balance

If you have had body image issues or are currently dealing with them, you may find it hard to understand what good balance looks like. If you struggle to avoid over-exercising, try to land on a level of exercise that makes you feel energised and motivated, but not so much that you're exhausted, pushing yourself too much or causing yourself physical or mental stress. If this is too much to unpick on your own, do seek professional help.

MOVEMENT DIARY

Write down how much you moved each day this week.

Monday:

Tuesday:

Wednesday:

Thursday:

Friday:

Saturday:

Sunday:

HEALTH ANXIETY

One area of anxiety that I am still learning about is health anxiety, which can easily turn to panic and chronic stress.

You'll remember that when we discussed stress and anxiety with Dr Jud earlier, we learned that anxiety doesn't have a clear precipitant like stress does. So if you are stressed about your health, it will probably be due to physical symptoms or a diagnosis, whereas health anxiety isn't always attached to symptoms or any diagnosed problems at all.

Recently, in an episode of our *Happy Place* YouTube series 'What Is, How To', I interviewed health anxiety expert Cherelle Roberts. She once suffered with debilitating health anxiety and now uses her training and experience to help others. She described symptoms that would lead to extreme fear, obsessive googling and multiple doctors' appointments. No level of reassurance would help convince her she was OK. Cherelle also experienced very real symptoms occurring from the attention she gave to certain worries. The stress she felt from this anxiety created actual health issues that reconfirmed Cherelle's fears. It's a complex form of anxiety, but one that's not impossible to overcome.

Interview with Alice Liveing

Personal trainer, author and app founder Alice Liveing has experienced health anxiety over the years and has talked about it openly. Let's find out more and get a better understanding of the stresses that might be causing her health anxiety and how the anxiety itself causes her stress.

Alice, tell me what your health anxiety feels like.

AL: For me, health anxiety is all-consuming. It's not just a fleeting feeling of a potential illness, it's a debilitating, unwavering worry that you're seriously unwell. I've had periods of my life where I've been at the doctors' multiple times in a week, convinced that they must have missed something and that I am in imminent danger. Oftentimes this anxiety comes out of nowhere and goes from nothing to unbearable in the space of a matter of hours.

Unlike other types of anxiety, which can often bubble under the surface, this anxiety throws my rational mind out of the window and takes hold of me in a way that I cannot even describe. It feels like I cannot do anything because I'm completely paralysed, in a state of fear.

Is it a constant anxiety or does it peak and trough?

It tends to peak and trough. The anxiety is always there, but sometimes it's fleeting thoughts like 'I've got a headache, I must have a brain tumour,' which I can then quickly rationalise and move on from, to 'I am dying.' And I cannot seem to make my brain believe I am not.

When it's at its worst, what thoughts are running through your head?

It's really the worst-case scenarios. Either that I'm dying, or that I have a debilitating chronic illness. It's as if my brain cannot think about anything other than this being the case. This is usually accompanied by symptom checking hundreds of times a day. Feeling my body for lumps, 'testing' myself in multiple ways and googling everything under the sun, which further exacerbates the issue.

How does that stress land in your body?

It usually feels like 'real' symptoms of whatever illness I feel I'm presenting with. That could be anything from chest pains, shortness of breath, dizziness, blurred vision, headaches, pins and needles, to muscle pains, fatigue, and more. These symptoms feel so visceral and real that they become debilitating and often stop me from doing anything other than focusing on them.

How do you come down from an episode?

At the moment my health anxiety is such that I need to see a doctor to help me come down from an episode. I wish I was at a point where I could independently rationalise that I am OK, but I'm just not there yet, so I spend a lot of time at the doctor getting tests and making sure I am actually OK.

I do have therapy alongside this and am undergoing a treatment called EMDR, which has good evidence to support it helping people with health anxiety, but it's definitely a work in process.

What helps you manage the stress of experiencing health anxiety?

Health anxiety for me is about control and it stems from childhood trauma. Being in control is something I feel I need, and a lack of control is often a trigger for health-related anxiety for me. While this is absolutely something I'm trying to work on, I do find that for now, keeping a good routine and doing all the things I know make me feel good – exercise, movement, sleep, good nutrition and social connection – do help me to avoid a big onset.

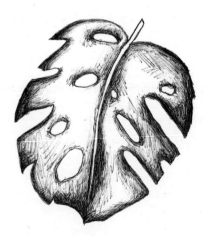

Little things that can help reduce health anxiety

❀ In our *Happy Place* YouTube episode, Cherelle Roberts explained that having only one chosen and reliable source of information online is imperative. Going down a Google rabbit hole can be extremely distressing, so pick one reliable online source, for example the NHS website, and stick to it.

❀ Therapy is sometimes necessary when it comes to recovering fully from anxiety. Therapy can be expensive and hard to come by, so you could look into charities that might be able to offer support.

❀ Check out the breathing technique that Cherelle offers in our YouTube episode. It's a technique that helps to calm the nervous system, so if you are spiralling into anxiety, it slows down the physical symptoms. It's two short, sharp breaths in and one long breath out.

❀ Also, take note of Alice's advice and see if you are keeping a routine that suits you – eating well, checking in with friends and moving when you can.

SOUL SICKNESS

I have to thank my friend Donna Lancaster for finding the right words to articulate the feeling I know many people experience, including me. 'Soul sickness' encompasses those times where you feel like the life has been sucked out of you. You might feel flat, lethargic and low without any specific cause. The meat of the feeling might be sadness, or even depression, but the side dish is most certainly a large portion of stress. The stress of not knowing why we feel so low; the tension of not experiencing enough joy and wondering why we are getting life wrong. I've certainly had moments where nothing seemed to make sense around me, and I severed all relations with joy. It's a really common feeling, but one we perhaps don't normally have the language for. Before Donna gifted me the phrase, I would have called this feeling an 'ick'.

This low-level stress might not have the fire of cortisol pumping and adrenaline surging, and it might not have the acidity of rage and injustice, but it's there. It's a dull hum that extracts your energy and lowers your optimism. In these moments it can be hard to decipher what exactly is causing the stress, so let's bypass that and work out how we can boost our joy and feed our soul.

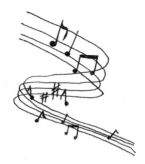

Little things to make your soul sing

❀ **Commit to meet up with a good friend once a week for coffee.** Remember Marc Schulz and Robert J. Waldinger's findings I mentioned earlier, about socialising? The more social contact we have, the more boosted we will feel, and the better long-term physical and mental health we will have.

❀ **Enjoy long walks** with beautiful music in your headphones.

❀ **Try painting.** Is there a local art club near you? My parents joined one a few years ago and it's given them so much joy.

❀ **Have small moments of awareness.** Many meditation teachers I have worked with at the Happy Place festivals and on our app have taught me about these important micro-moments. Each day you could set an alarm and then spend the next two minutes just focusing on what you can smell, hear, see, taste and feel. These moments of awareness get us out of relentless rumination and more into the now.

❀ **Support one another.** One of the easiest ways we can feed our souls is to help someone else. Support a friend or a relative in need, or you could sign up to local programmes to help those in need in your area. Even just texting a friend who is having a tough time or sending a handwritten card to show you love them will improve your mood.

❀ **Writing.** Why not start a daily or weekly diary? Feel free to get out any negative feelings you have onto the page but also include what you're thankful for. Start up a list of dreams and desires and make mood boards to help you move towards the things that make you feel joyful.

❀ **Listen to interesting stories on podcasts or in audiobooks.** Make sure you're choosey about what you listen to. Does it leave you feeling light and bright, or fearful and low? Go with audio that leaves you feeling better than before.

❀ **Try something new.** It doesn't have to be wildly scary or out of the ordinary; it could simply be starting up a conversation with someone in your local café for the first time, or switching up what you would normally eat for lunch. Experiencing newness encourages us to be mentally flexible, giving us a greater propensity to challenge ourselves and grow.

Connect and create

I have always found creativity to be a shortcut to feeling boosted and alive. Even if you don't see yourself as a creative person, there is a huge opportunity for more art and invention in your life. I'm much more creative than I am academic. My brain is a constant whirr of ideas that I feel desperate to execute. I love nothing more than to paint, write poems, conjure up ideas, build, create boards on Pinterest and brainstorm. The gratitude I feel for that creativity is off the scale; it's my crutch when I am feeling low. Explore creative endeavours with friends and family members, in online communities and in your local area. It's a real balm for the soul, cultivates connection and subsequently helps with physical and mental stress reduction.

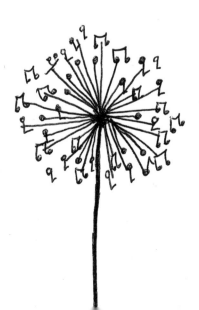

WHAT MAKES YOUR SOUL SING?

1

2

3

4

5

6

7

8

This week, try to engage with at least one of the soul boosters on your list. Rather than scrolling on your phone, call that mate for a catch-up. On weekends when you don't have plans, do that hobby that makes you feel zingy. Do what makes you feel good, lessen that low hum of stress and make your soul sing.

AWESTRUCK

One of the reasons many of us feel flat and soul-sick in adulthood is because we lose the knack for spotting moments of awe. As tiny kids we sit and watch a row of ants marching, with big wide eyes and minds full of wonder, and we look up at the night skies with millions of questions. When we move into adulthood, we don't spot the ants or bother to look up at the stars overhead. We become jaded to the wonders that are all around us.

I went on a run yesterday and because I've currently got awe on the brain, I made sure to look around me to tune into it. On the side of the road, amongst a scrappy patch of grass, stood a tall, elegant, dusty pink poppy. The colour was the most delicious shade of pink I've ever seen. I could have very easily run straight past that poppy and instead focused on the list of to-dos in my scattered mind. We must retrain our brains to spot wonder and create a new habit of doing so.

When we see the world through childlike eyes, we can spot the beauty and wonder around us and feel more connected, curious and hopefully less stressed.

Mindfulness has been practised for thousands of years in different guises, and the word has been batted around a lot in the last decade due to our increased interest in wellness. You might have read about it in a book, or heard it mentioned on a podcast, but still not really have a solid idea about what it is. Mindfulness is simply the act of being fully conscious of what you're doing, whether that's sitting quietly with your thoughts and observing the world around you or working on a task that has your full attention. You might already be practising mindfulness without realising it. It's really not that complicated. It should be an activity or practice that allows a steady, cool concentration, so your mind rarely wanders, and one that makes you feel open rather than closed, as Dr Jud discussed at the start of the book. A feeling of openness is one where we feel connected, alive and buoyant.

My friend, the yoga teacher Zephyr Wildman, thinks the term 'mindfulness' can be misleading, as we are actually trying to cultivate a less full mind, so she often uses the term 'awakefulness' in her yoga classes. My own version of mindfulness/awakefulness would be painting or drawing. The fluid motion of a brush on canvas, or the delicate touch of pencil to paper, is enough to slow down time, erase racing thoughts and bring me fully into the present. Any activity that calms the nervous system and allows you to focus on one given task can sit under the heading of mindfulness.

Don't worry if you still find your mind racing or jumping from random thought to random thought. Just being aware that your mind is racing is a good start. We're looking for awareness here, not a completely blank mind.

What mindful activity do you already practise?

....

How does it make you feel?

....

How often do you do it?

....

Could you do it more often?

....

If you don't yet have one, what activity do you think would be enjoyable?

....

LAUGH OUT LOUD

When you're stressed, one of the first things to go out of the window is your sense of humour. We turn to catastrophising and fail to see the funny side of life. My disclaimer here is that of course there are many stressful things that are not funny whatsoever, but in some situations, there is room for humour.

I recently interviewed comedian and activist Fats Timbo, who was raised in a family that prioritises humour. Their trip to Tenerife is beautifully demonstrative of this as the entire family missed their flight home by a day and chose to laugh hysterically for half an hour straight. Fats's retelling of this story on my podcast hit me like a brick. I know that in a similar situation I would have flapped, wept a bit and chosen stress over humour. I think back to Fats's story whenever I know I'm not seeing the funny side of life. Finding the humour in life is a habit we can cultivate. We can practise choosing to see another angle and look for the laughter.

When was the last time you really laughed? Whenever I'm with my oldest mates I regress to being about 14 and end up in fits of giggles. We met for dinner recently and my face ached from laughing afterwards.

After that dinner I felt buoyed for weeks. It sparked an inner mischievousness where I found myself hunting down the next thing that could make me howl. Everything seemed a little funnier and a lot less serious. It seems laughter breeds laughter.

Who or what makes you laugh the most?

. . . .

. . . .

. . . .

This week, aim to spend time with that person or watch that TV show that makes you laugh out loud. It's the most fun way to reduce stress in the mind and body.

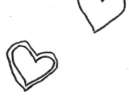

CONTROL

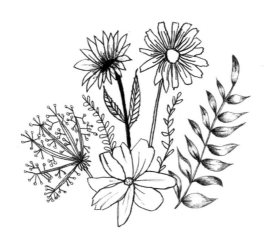

So much of the stress we experience comes from a lack of control, or our attempts to try to gain it. Feeling out of control makes me very stressed and brings out the worst in me. I like visual order, lists, a schedule of what is happening when and where, piles of neatly stacked life admin, folded clothes. My friends and family often comment on how disciplined I am in my routine; I'm like clockwork when it comes to how my day pans out, even amid an ever-changing schedule and varying working hours. What my nearest and dearest don't see is that I create order, routine and structure to feel safe and less stressed. Without my morning coffee made in exactly the same way each day, or my bedtime routine with its multitude of idiosyncrasies, I feel like I'm falling apart. As soon as I start to feel the wheels coming off, my stress levels skyrocket. Yet at times I realise that this rigidity is stopping me from experiencing newness and isn't helping me become mentally flexible, which is so needed when it comes to stress reduction.

Let's face it, life is often uncontrollable – from the weather to how other people behave, to global events and systemic problems – so there will always be stress. How well we cope in unexpected moments, and how we respond to stress, is the only part of the deal we have control over. Some of us find safety in creating control in our everyday lives, whereas others feel more at ease with the unexpected. Some of this will be due to our upbringing and what was modelled to us, as well as the challenges we have previously faced in life.

Do you find yourself attempting to micromanage every step of the day, to feel more in control? Or do you feel more at home in the unexpected? Write down your thoughts below.

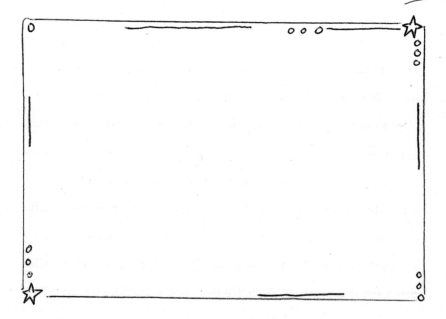

FAMILY TREE PATTERNS

Often the way in which we react to life's twists and turns reflects what we have picked up from our parents.

There are always going to be questions around the nature vs nurture debate, but I'm fairly sure most of us can see how our own behaviour mirrors what we have seen growing up. My mum came on to the *Happy Place* podcast as a guest last year to discuss generational patterns. It gave me the space to ask questions I hadn't before, and I learned a lot about my mum and nan. My mum's mum, Sylvia, suffered with depression and anxiety throughout my mum's childhood. She had given birth to my mum at the age of 18 and throughout Mum's early life would regularly visit a psychiatric day ward. My nan's mood was often unpredictable, so Mum was left confused at times. My dear nan's mental health had been compromised by the acute pain she had experienced in the war. As a child during the Second World War, she was evacuated out of London to stay with an abusive woman in Wales, and around this time lost her sister to TB. Her trauma was unprocessed and unhealed, and her mental health suffered greatly. On the podcast, Mum also talked about my grandad's anxiety. He was overly cautious about safety, which led to obsessive lock checking, multiple locks on doors, and getting my mum and aunty to practise what to do if they were in a motorway car crash. Mum's childhood has informed how she reacts to stress today. I have full empathy for what my family members endured, without judgement, and I can also see how these patterns have leaked into my own life. Picking up family traits and reactions to stress can feel unavoidable.

Can you see patterns of behaviour in your own family background that may have contributed to how you react to moments where you feel out of control? Write a little about this below, and if you feel it would be helpful and think it's achievable, could you instigate a conversation with members of your family who could piece together the puzzle?

....

....

....

....

....

Little things to help break the patterns of stress

❄ **Trace back to where these patterns began.** Look at how your mum and dad, or carers growing up, reacted to stress. There doesn't need to be any blame or resentment here; each generation has done their best to cope. These patterns might have formed many generations back. Then remember this is learned behaviour which can subsequently be unlearned. It might not be easy to unpick years of ingrained behaviour but there is always room for movement. Having the awareness that it's a learned pattern is a very good start.

❄ **Get curious about how and when you started to use these learned behaviours as your own coping mechanisms.** When we are curious about our own behaviours and patterns, we take the heat and self-judgement out of the equation. Nobody needs self-loathing on top of the stress.

❄ **Notice your reaction.** Next time you catch yourself reacting to stress in a habitual way, rather than immediately trying to change that reaction, just notice how you feel. Has that habitual reaction made you feel angry, out of control, righteous, scared, or victimised? When I'm stressed, I feel as if my world is crumbling around me. It feels like everything is going wrong, which is often disproportionate to what I'm actually experiencing. Being able to pinpoint the feelings breaks down the process a little. Just noticing these feelings is enough to begin with. If we start by wanting instant change, we may give up when we don't see immediate results.

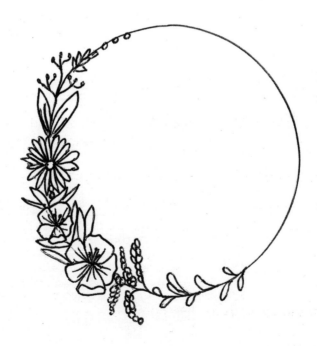

PHOBIAS AND FEARS

Generational trauma, or past pain in your own life, can lead to phobias. Whether it's snakes, spiders, small spaces, motorways, flying, heights or the sea, the manifestation of this fear can appear in many forms. The difference between a phobia and a fear is that fear is a normal reaction to something scary or dangerous, whereas a phobia leads to an acute fear response even when you might not be in danger.

Therapies that can help lessen the stress of phobias are exposure therapy, which exposes you to your phobia to help you gain control, and CBT (Cognitive Behavioural Therapy). CBT can also effectively reduce anxiety, help with phobias, PTSD, tics and depression, and is used as a means of treatment for substance abuse. It helps challenge thoughts and beliefs and associated behaviours to improve emotional regulation. Another option to consider is somatic therapy, which focuses on what is going on in the mind and body and how the two work together. It can include breathwork, meditation, shaking the body, dance, massage and other forms of body movement. Somatic work helps target muscle memory and tension and stress in the body, so we can create new neural pathways and form new habits.

These are just a few types of effective therapy you could research further, if they resonate. If you feel debilitated by your phobias, I would highly recommend getting professional help, as these therapies can be remarkably effective. But there are still simple ways to help you manage and cope with the stress of experiencing phobias.

Little things you can do to reduce phobia-related stress

❀ **Remember that it's possible to overcome phobias.** When I went through a period of being terrified of motorways, I honestly felt there would never be a way out. I landed on acceptance that I would never drive on a motorway again. Giving up on any hope felt easier than facing this phobia head on. For five years I felt down about it, and quite stressed when I had to turn down family get-togethers or visiting friends. I'm here to remind you it is possible to overcome these big fears, as I can now drive on the motorway relatively stress-free. I sometimes feel a small twinge of fear creep in, but I am now able to push it to one side to get on with my journey. I'm naturally an anxious person, so if I can do it, you definitely can.

❀ **Say your fears out loud.** When we bury thoughts, they seem a lot bigger and scarier than they need to be. The mere thought of a motorway would make me feel sick, so my attempt at controlling these feelings was to bury them. I would push the fear to the bottom of my thoughts and ignore the feelings, rather than get curious about them. Over time I realised it was important to honour those feelings so I could get to know them better. I needed to say aloud, 'I am terrified I'm going to faint on the motorway and have a fatal car crash.' That was my root fear and one I needed to challenge. Without admitting my worst thoughts, I could not heal from them.

❀ **Go easy on yourself.** Overcoming phobias can take years but it's worth trying. The long road is better than being static and crushed by your phobia. Slowly and gently always; there is no rush at all.

❀ **Mark your progress in a journal.** Two years ago I took a friend with me onto the M4 and managed a twenty-minute journey at the wheel. I had pangs of panic, but those feelings didn't progress into a full-blown panic attack. It felt like a huge moment and gave me a lot of confidence to try again. Marking these moments down allows you to track how you are incrementally progressing.

✻ **Speak to others who are going through something similar.** I have since met so many people who share that same phobia of motorways, which has made me feel much less alone. It's easy to feel like you are the only one experiencing the stress of a particular phobia, but you are never alone.

HABITS

Humans are creatures of habit, with our days linked together by a series of familiar activities. Some of these habits are beneficial, such as cleaning our teeth. Some habits are benign, like drinking a cup of coffee every day or walking a certain route to work, and some are detrimental, like smoking, excessive drinking or binge eating. Good habits often take time to establish, as we must repeat the action over and over until our brains see it as beneficial. For example, if we want to create a new habit of exercising, we have to put effort in to begin with and stick to it for a few weeks for the habit to form. The initial period of forming a good habit takes willpower and effort but then, over time, our brains get used to the idea and the amount of effort needed lessens. Our brains need that repetition and some conclusive proof to keep it up. If we start to notice that we feel mentally and physically better than before, we will feel more motivated to stick to it.

When I interviewed Jason Derulo for the *Happy Place* podcast recently, he gave me some very grounded advice when it comes to sticking to good habits. He cites routine as being the making of him, because he believes it takes the emotion out of the equation. He says that a routine means you just do the thing every day whether you want to or not. You don't leave brushing your teeth one morning because you don't feel like it.

Unfortunately, when it comes to bad habits we don't need to put quite so much effort in at the start. Detrimental habits are often a knee-jerk reaction to stress, pain, discomfort, boredom or overwhelm. Our brains want out and a bad habit allows us to momentarily bypass whatever we do not want to feel.

If we are incredibly stressed, we might pick up our phones and scroll through endless photos on social media, to instantly numb the feeling and distract us. If we are overwhelmed at work, we may reach for a bag of sugary sweets to comfort ourselves. In these moments of stress, we usually turn to detrimental habits rather than positive ones, as they take a lot less effort. We also tend to ignore or learn to live with the subsequent side effects of such habits. We get used to the hangovers, or bad cough or mental fog, and the urge to lean back into that bad habit overrides the worry or pain we subsequently experience. You might find yourself momentarily numbing stress by drinking, smoking, using your phone excessively, binge eating, online shopping, gambling or restricting your food intake. It could even be as simple as bitching about people. There are of course much more extreme detrimental habits in times of stress, such as bulimia, self-harm, drug use and so on, which are likely to need professional guidance to break.

For many years, when I was triggered by stress I would purge. It became a crutch I would use when my life felt out of control, yet ironically the habit kept me in a loop of feeling even more out of control. Bulimia is often much more than a bad habit. It's classed as a mental illness and an eating disorder, but part of the action for me was completely habitual. It was familiar and offered a vague promise of safety. I later learned there was truly little safety with this technique of seeking relief and I was luckily able to heal and recover.

Do you have any detrimental habits that you turn to when you're stressed?

....

....

....

....

How do you think this habit negatively impacts you?

....

....

....

....

Sometimes, when I'm feeling stressed, I will use social media to escape the feelings I'm experiencing. As I mindlessly scroll through photos of distant beaches I'm not on and make-up tutorials I will never recreate, I distract myself from the stress I'm feeling. The thing is, after slipping into this mental oblivion, I actually end up feeling worse.

Let's revisit Dr Jud's words from earlier. He taught us that if we feel the urge to fall into a negative habitual pattern, we can take a pause. Rather than instantly picking up the cigarette, phone or glass of wine, we can sit with the feeling of discomfort. Try it. We are all addicted to our phones and devices, so the next time you feel the urge to check your emails, scroll on social media or check a news site, pause. Feel the sensation the urge brings. It might be discomfort, a burst of energy, irritation or restlessness. Just be with it. It might not feel nice, but it cannot harm us.

How did the pause make you feel? What came up?

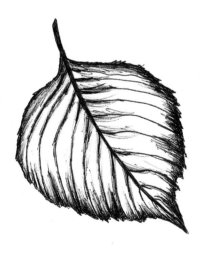

. . . .

. . . .

. . . .

. . . .

Little things to help ride out an urge

❀ **Pause and breathe.** Focus on your inhale and exhale. Even if it's just for ten breaths. A small moment of mindfulness will help calm your nervous system and recalibrate your thoughts.

❀ **Get curious about the stress you are feeling.** What is it you are trying to escape?

❀ **Be compassionate.** Self-compassion is imperative so you don't slip into self-loathing. Your stress is valid. There will always be someone out there in an even more stressful situation, but that doesn't mean you can't accept and experience your own feelings. Feel them, get curious about them and practise self-compassion.

❀ **Think about how you will feel after reaching for your bad habit.** As well as momentary relief, will you also feel drained? Or low? Or filled with self-loathing?

❀ **Replace the bad habit will another action.** Could you go for a short walk? Listen to music? Or write down how you feel?

❀ **Chart your progress.** Keep a log of how you are doing and don't feel defeated if you don't manage to break the chain of the negative habit straight away. If you have a day where you slip up, don't worry. Even lessening the detrimental habit is great progress.

❀ **Find a buddy to go on this journey with you.** If you have a friend or relative who is equally keen to break a detrimental habit, partner up with them to cheerlead each other and be there in the tougher moments. They don't even need to share the same habit; they just need to be on board with attempting to make positive changes.

❀ **Some changes in behaviour will require navigating other people's questions.** I stopped drinking for about a year in my thirties and was constantly questioned when out at parties or weddings. I met this line of questioning with a practised response. I explained that I was feeling the benefits of not drinking, and then I would change the subject. Peer pressure doesn't help when you're trying to give up a detrimental habit. You might encounter others who want you to partake in their smoking, drinking, binge eating or gossiping because it makes them feel better to have someone else along for the ride. This is where you really need to lean into the pause and think back to your reasons for making this change.

❀ **Talk to someone about how you are feeling.** If you are really struggling to break a detrimental habit, get honest with someone. Talk to a friend or relative about the emotions behind the habit. Do you feel scared? Alone? Out of control? Saying it aloud really does take the heat out of the issue. When I started out on my healing journey to recover from bulimia, I found it exceedingly difficult to say the words out loud. I knew I felt scared and out of control but I also felt embarrassed to talk about it. Luckily, over time and with practice, I can now talk about that part of my life with ease. I don't feel embarrassed at all; if anything it has offered me a connection with others who have experienced something similar. If you don't feel able to talk about these feelings with someone, try saying the words out loud to yourself. Even hearing your own voice articulating the feelings takes the secrecy and shame out of the equation.

PRAYER

I'm not religious, nor do I pray to a particular god or goddess, but I constantly seek spiritual connection. Non-religious prayer is an act of handing over control to something bigger than us, and we don't have to align with one certain doctrine to do it. Surrendering in a moment of stress and asking for help or guidance can be a huge comfort.

A non-religious prayer can be spoken aloud, and a moment where you ask for support or guidance. Don't get too hung up on who you are talking to. You might want to ask the universe, the spirit of a deceased loved one, or keep it totally ambiguous. Conversely, that something that is bigger than us is also within us, therefore you can ask your heart for guidance and support. You might want to write the prayer in a notebook or just think it in your head. There are no rules. You just need to ask for the guidance. Praying doesn't mean the answer reveals itself immediately, but you might notice a lessening of stress, a feel of support, and down the line new thoughts, or ideas.

I believe it's important that we don't exclusively use prayer in times of stress but also when we want to offer up gratitude or simply speak our thoughts aloud. The more we pray, the more natural it feels to do so, no matter how we are feeling. Pray for help, guidance, gratitude, or whatever feels natural to you.

It may seem as if there has been a new surge of interest in spirituality, but having spiritual beliefs or faith is one of the oldest stress busters out there. If you already align with a certain religion, you'll have your own set of outlines and methods in which to pray, but if not just try experimenting to work out what feels right to you.

In times of great stress, we may pray for a positive outcome. We may ask for our health to improve, or for a loved one to be OK. There is of course nothing wrong with this and we may experience good outcomes, but there is never a guarantee. When I am stressed or going through a challenging time, I prefer to pray to be guided through it. I ask for help in navigating tough times and for the strength to move through them as peacefully as possible. This puts the emphasis on my response to the stress rather than the situation itself. Praying always makes me feel that bit lighter, as if the stress has been diluted.

Have you ever prayed?

YES   NO

control

Write down a little prayer here if you feel you need guidance. There are no rules: just write freely and ask for what you need.

LOOKING OUTSIDE

One of the everyday factors that we have absolutely no control over is how others perceive us. I have felt enormous amounts of stress caused by my worry about what others think of me. In my line of work, it's inevitable, and although I've been in the public eye since the age of 15, I still find it desperately uncomfortable. You might therefore wonder why I am still in it. If I find it so irksome, why haven't I found a job that allows me anonymity and less stress? Sometimes I ask myself this very question, but I love my job so much it's a downside I'm willing to endure for now.

Perversely, I also quite like the challenge of managing this stress. Being in the public eye and having no control over how others perceive me forces me to drop my ego and let go. I cannot be too tied to who I believe I am and how others should see me. There is a beautiful Ram Dass quote that says, *'It's really time to see through the absurdity of your own predicament, you aren't who you thought you were.'* Who we think we are, or what others have told us we are, is only a tiny fraction of the truth or someone else's opinion. Being curious about who you are is one of the most expansive and exciting mindsets we can have.

We must also remember that whenever anyone verbally attacks or criticises us it has nothing to do with us and everything to do with them. Next time you experience negative outside judgement, see if you can detect the other person's pain underneath their words. Those who overly criticise, verbally attack or judge others are people in pain. A happy, self-content person wouldn't have the need.

Little things to limit stress from outside judgement

Don't add your own judgement to the equation. It is unhelpful to start judging yourself, on top of the outside opinions you're dealing with. Seek self-compassion. It's in there somewhere, even if it feels hard to locate. Start by honouring the parts of yourself that feel broken or hurt and let whatever emotion flow that needs to.

Do not abandon yourself. When I would read hurtful online comments or nasty press stories about myself in the past, my initial reaction was always to abandon myself. I believed that I deserved negative feedback and told myself I was worthless. Now, I know better and vow to have my own back and stand by what I know to be true – that I'm a good person with good intentions. I will get things wrong, have flaws, slip up and speak without thinking at times, but inherently I am a good person who deserves to be stood by and not abandoned.

Notice the other person's/people's pain. Why are they firing abuse, judgement or negative opinions your way? What is it inside them that's hurting?

Remember, we have no control over how others see us. If we waste energy trying to manipulate how others see us we will end up acting inauthentically, feeling drained and disconnected from who we really are. The only thing you can do is be YOU.

Noticing and celebrating the parts of ourselves we like builds a strong foundation when it comes to the outside world's opinion of us. Add to the list of things you like about yourself whenever you want. You may find over time you become more accepting of, or even fall in love with, parts of yourself you didn't even know existed.

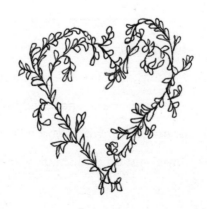

MONEY

I rarely feel comfortable talking about money. My buttocks are clenching as I enter this section of the book. I don't think many people do like discussing it, but I believe women especially struggle with this one. There is an awkwardness about it and each one of us will have a very different relationship with money. It may have caused you immense amounts of stress over the years, have tarnished your childhood, or have given you freedom. It's a huge, complicated subject and one that many feel is out of their control. And of course, at times it is. Again, what we do have control over is our emotional response to money.

Below, write down what your reaction to financial stress feels like.

....

....

....

....

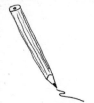

Did you learn this reaction in childhood? Did your parents or carers have a certain narrative around money during your childhood? What did you learn about money as a kid?

....

....

....

Equality and fairness

We may have fears, hatred, or confusion around money due to our upbringing, but if we can trace back to where those ideas formed we have a chance to un-learn what we've picked up. There are of course systemic prejudices when it comes to pay, with data highlighting that discrimination is still rife when it comes to equal pay for women, people of colour, the LGBTQ+ community and the disability community. This disparity is unfortunately a massive barrier for so many when it comes to income and financial security. These barriers can't be ignored as progress is imperative. There is also still a ginormous lack of support when it comes to working mothers and single parents, which can lead to immense stress and fewer opportunities. These are huge issues that we don't have full control over, but one thing we do control is our attitude towards money. Sometimes without even realising it we become used to what we are told in childhood or by society today. We might devalue ourselves in the workplace and feel we are undeserving of a promotion, pay rise or new opportunities.

Do you believe you deserve opportunities, promotions, a crack at your own business or pay rises?

....

....

Money blocks often stem from a place of self-esteem. Our self-esteem issues within the context of our financial lives may have been formed in childhood, or due to a sour work situation as well as generation patterns and systemic barriers as part of a minority. If you have grown up understanding your caregivers were under financial stress or have been told repeatedly that you do not and will not have enough, then you may have a block in this area. You may have heard a parent comment on how little money was around in your childhood and that has led to you believing the same. You may have been sacked, made redundant or told you were failing at work, which has led to a lack of confidence in this area. When our confidence gets knocked it can feel very tricky to find the energy to build it back up and try again, but it is not impossible.

On the opposite page, write down a list of your best professional assets that you value. It could be your kindness, your willingness to work hard, creativity, problem solving, work ethic or a specific skill set.

Look back on this list and always remember your worth. The more you focus on it, the more others will see it.

Putting a price on your work when self-employed can feel embarrassing and awkward, yet you're the only one who can determine that price. It may take time to establish your worth in a new area of work, but your level of experience and skill set should set the tone. If you have the experience, something unique or helpful to offer, or a skill set you have honed, don't be embarrassed to declare your worth. If you are an employee and believe a pay rise is appropriate this is also something you may consider asking for. Look back on your list and remember your worth.

MY SKILLS AND ASSETS

1 ....

2 ....

3 ....

4 ....

5 ....

6 ....

7 ....

8 ....

WORK IT

Powerlessness in the workplace is the cause of catastrophic stress for so many. We might feel out of control because we're on the first rung of our career ladder, or feel like we're undermined creatively, intellectually or otherwise by colleagues. Maybe we don't agree with the values of the workplace we find ourselves in, or don't like the job itself. It took me twenty years to feel like I had control in my working life, which I hope is empowering to hear rather than daunting.

The twenty-odd years of my career prior to founding my brand Happy Place were a roller coaster. Obviously they weren't all bad, but I spent a lot of time feeling utterly out of control. Step back with me to the year 1996, where a young girl from the suburbs of London who has just had her braces removed walks onto the set of a kids' TV show for the first time. There is a slight expectation that I should know how it all works; that I'll have a level of comfort in front of the looming cameras. I'm excited, enthralled, but utterly petrified. I spent many years after this moment feeling exactly the same. I longed to feel comfortable and look like I belonged.

A few years down the line in my career, the pendulum swayed in the other direction as I started to disengage with what was going on around me in order to cope. As I discussed earlier, the way I attempted to reduce stress and gain control was through bulimia, people-pleasing and exaggerating my personality. For much of the twenty years I was on TV I felt I had little control over my work. I would be given a script, autocue and earpiece, and direction as to how I should perform. There was also huge pressure to look a certain way, whether that be my physical body or how I dressed. My personality on screen was reduced to about 20 per cent of who I really was.

There were happy times and extraordinary moments – I met people I hugely admired and travelled all over the world – but I didn't feel I had much control at all. Then a set of circumstances that were extremely mentally challenging entered the scene, which led to a whack of depression. During this period, I ended up leaving the jobs that made me feel the most restricted. I was grateful for those jobs, but I also needed to be free of them. I jumped out of the plane into nothingness, with no direction or safety net.

The best part of my new career, my second chance, as I like to call it, is that I have more control. I cannot be sacked, told what to wear, how to speak, or which subjects to discuss. It's taken a lot of work and dedication but I'm much happier now I feel I'm steering the ship. That's not to say I don't experience stress in my new line of work. The pressure of building and running a multifaceted company often leads to overwhelm and exhaustion, but I believe it's worth it, as I'm hugely passionate about the work I'm doing.

Do you feel out of control at work?

....

....

Why is that? Who or what is controlling your working life?

....

....

....

....

Little things to give you more control at work

❀ **Make work a happy space.** If you don't like your job but know it isn't possible to change it right now, can you look at the relationships you have there? Is there one or more person/s that you connect with daily? Improving our relationships at work creates a much happier experience and gives us the opportunity to take back control of our stress levels. Creating healthy relationships at work requires effort. Gravitate towards the people who make you feel boosted and set boundaries with those that don't.

❀ **Look for your purpose.** The word *purpose* can sound a little pretentious and grand, but it doesn't have to be that way. Finding your purpose might not be as drastic as creating systemic change or saving lives; it might just be brightening the days of those around you.

❀ **Speak up when you have an idea.** If you currently feel invisible at work and undervalued, make yourself heard. Speaking up can feel exposing, as there's no guarantee that your ideas will land, but it is still absolutely worth it. The more we flex that muscle, the easier it becomes, and the better we get at handling rejection if our ideas are not wanted.

❀ **Control your own space.** If you feel out of control at work because you're bored, then look for interests outside of work to gain some balance. When I felt particularly disengaged at work, I would paint all evening when I got home. It was not only an amazing stress reliever; it also made me feel alive and connected.

❀ **Dare to dream.** We might feel we are being foolish to dream about other opportunities. As children we are constantly asked, 'What would you like to be when you're older?' We are encouraged to dream big. We might say we want to be an astronaut, a ballet dancer or a scientist. Do not feel silly about dreaming big. What is it that you really want to do? Life is short; too short to be hating a job that has you in its grip for hours at a time.

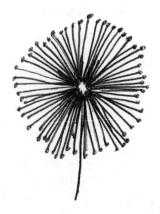

PERFECTION

Perfectionism is the sneakiest of traits. Without you even realising it, it'll be blocking you in so many ways and causing stress in places you are yet to discover. Striving for perfection is a common way to seek out control, in the hope that carrying out a task or project to the highest of standards will make us feel complete. The terrible news is: there is no completion. There is no moment where any of us step back and can say, 'Yes, I have reached utter perfection.' Even international athletes, whose main career objective is to have moments of perfection in order to get that gold medal, cannot mitigate fear, self-doubt, or stress in the long term.

We might also use perfectionism to protect ourselves. I suffer with this enormously. Having spoken with many a brilliant brain I can now see with more clarity that my need for perfection is a form of safeguarding from imagined future disaster. Making sure that my kitchen utensils are all facing the same way will not stop me from getting a parking ticket later that day. Producing the perfect episode of my podcast, *Happy Place*, will not negate my kids having a massive homework meltdown. Ironically, striving for perfection to mitigate stress actually causes a lot more stress. It is not only draining and time consuming but also usually leads to resentment. If we are not careful perfectionism can lead to total burnout; a subject I cover in more depth later on in the book.

Little things to help with letting go of perfect

❁ **Look at what you have learned from the messier parts of life.** Maybe in the past you've experienced a break-up or messed up at work. There is always something to learn from moments that are less than ideal. There are many more lessons in the mess than in the perfect.

❁ **Give yourself a break.** None of us perform perfectly every day. Some days we need to just be average, or less than average. Sometimes we need rest, to keep ourselves in balance. There is not a single person on the planet who is getting everything right.

❁ **Next time you catch yourself striving for perfection, check in with your stress levels.** What do you believe will happen if you are not perfect? Do you believe you'll be rejected? Told off? Shamed? Get to know those underlying beliefs and challenge them, because they aren't always true.

❁ **Celebrate your quirks.** My God, the world would be boring if everyone was perfect and getting it right all of the time. Champion the parts of you that are unique to you, whether you believe they're perfect or not. Your brilliant face, the words you accidently stutter, your idiosyncrasies, your quirky habits – you are bloody perfect as you are.

❁ **Don't be fooled into thinking that there's a future version of you that is perfect.** And don't be fooled into thinking you'll feel any happier when you achieve this supposed perfection. That is a horrendous loop to find ourselves in. Accepting who we are today is a much quicker way to drop the stress.

❁ **Allow yourself to be imperfect.** Sit with the feelings of discomfort about the parts of you, or your life, that you find challenging; but don't abandon those parts. It is OK for things to be a little bit messy, or sometimes extremely messy.

❁ **Remember: perfect cannot save us.**

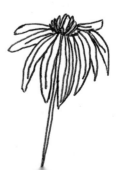

THE JUGGLE

Like some of you reading this, I'm a working mum. The pressure society places on the shoulders of working mothers causes a great deal of stress. We are supposed to raise perfect kids, who eat perfectly, speak perfectly, behave perfectly, sleep perfectly and do well at school. We are one of the first generations of women to have the opportunity to be CEOs, leaders, business founders, managers and to have careers. We not only have to work incredibly hard to prove ourselves in these new spaces, but to also carve a path for generations to come. Oh, and by the way, all while maintaining a social life.

FUCK THAT! It is impossible for any of us to be nailing it all. For those of you who are single parents, this pressure will be even more all-consuming. To attempt such a feat is going to cause insurmountable stress, burnout and a feeling of being utterly defeated. I recently watched an incredible talk by Shonda Rhimes, the American screenwriter, producer and author. Her rallying speech had me on my feet cheering at my phone screen from miles away in London. Her admission that every time she is nailing it at work, she is missing out on story time with her kids at home, and every time she is sewing a Halloween costume for her children, she is falling behind at work, made me feel much less alone in the pressure put upon women, or single parents. We simply cannot do it all.

Little things to take the pressure off

These days I like to think of my life as a pie chart. There is only one me and one you, so how we choose to split our time is vital if we want to reduce stress levels and lighten our load. My pie chart looks a little like this these days.

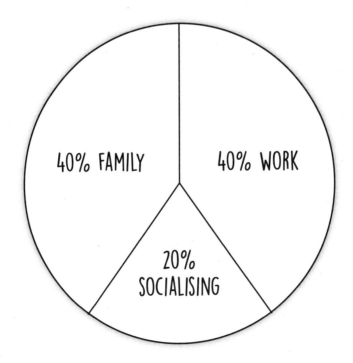

I have actively decided that my priorities are family and work. Yours might differ: there is no right or wrong here. If you don't have children, are single, do not work or otherwise, simply split the pie to see where your priorities currently sit. Your priorities might be your caring for someone, your spiritual life, your physical wellbeing or a hobby. Make the pie totally bespoke to you and your life. The chart is an effective way to see how much you are trying to cram in. If you are aiming for 100 per cent effort at work, 100 per cent in your family life and 100 per cent with your social scene, how is that going to fit in the pie? It isn't, and if you try to squeeze it all in there you are going to feel overwhelmed and stressed to the max. Divide your pie up on the page opposite.

This chart does not need to be set in stone. In the future your priorities may change as your life evolves, with changes in work, starting a family or your kids getting older. Just use it as a template to see where you want your attention to sit.

MY PIE CHART

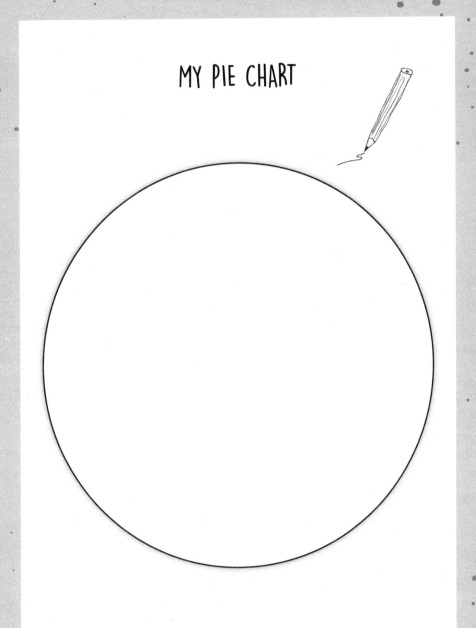

FERTILITY

This is a huge area that is more deserving of a whole book than one small chapter on stress. If this part of the book leaves you wanting more, please do check out www.ivfbabble.com for information and a true sense of community, Gabrielle Bernstein's conversations around fertility and Elizabeth Day's articles and books. There are so many brilliant women talking about fertility and forging community along the way.

If you have struggled with your fertility or are currently experiencing the stress from this challenging journey, then you will be sick of people telling you that stress is the worst thing when trying to conceive. Undoubtedly, your stress levels will rise even further with the pressure of now having to be completely relaxed, when you already feel out of control. That sort of advice is not beneficial at all. It's often a time when you feel broken, defeated and on edge as you play the waiting game.

Interview with Amanda

My cousin-in-law (is that a thing? You get the gist, my cousin's wife) Amanda has been on a fertility roller coaster over the last decade and is willing to share some insights on stress with us.

Amanda, tell us a little bit about your fertility journey.

A: It all started around 2014 when I was 32. I came off contraception with the idea that we'd fall pregnant before or after our wedding, which was set for July 2015.

After two years I knew something must be up, so I went to my doctor. I was referred for further tests with a gynaecologist and was diagnosed with hypothyroidism (underactive thyroid), anaemia and stage 4 (severe) endometriosis. I was eventually referred for IVF on the NHS at almost 35 years old. We were extremely lucky to be referred for IVF on the NHS and even luckier that the first round was successful and resulted in our little boy, who was born in May 2018.

Life with our little boy was everything we had imagined and more, but we always knew we wanted to add to our family and give him a sibling, and this time we knew that we were on our own, without the help of the NHS. We saved up and had our second round of IVF in early 2021. We went into it naively thinking it would work first time, because it had previously. But we were three years older, and this time it wasn't to be. It took three more rounds to get pregnant. Fast-forward to January 2023 and as I'm typing this I'm 29 weeks pregnant with a little baby boy on the way at 40 years old.

How stress-inducing has it all been?

It's not been an easy journey. Early on, I didn't handle news of other people's pregnancies well, especially ones that were close to home. This left me feeling guilty that I didn't want to be around all the joyous news, when it was all my family could talk about. I think Jess [Amanda's husband] struggled to know how to support me through this; it was no one's fault, but it definitely caused stress for us both while we navigated grieving a life we had longed for. All the while we were trying to put on our happy faces to celebrate with close family members, when it seemed like their good news had come easier for them.

Then you throw in work and the usual stress of day-to-day life. Working for a busy, fast-paced fashion retailer has its own challenges. With the first round of IVF I managed to do it all in private using my holidays, but I decided to have an honest conversation with my work when it came to my second and then third, fourth and fifth rounds. They were really support-ive and gave me time off to rest during the two-week wait of each round, although once I returned to work it was back to the normality of long days and constant meetings.

What is the most stressful aspect of trying to conceive through IVF?

The most stressful part is the fact that it feels completely out of your control, which it mostly is. But after the last round I realised there were some aspects we could take control of, which gave me some comfort. Each round left me feeling anxious – would it work, would this one end how previous rounds had? I'd analyse every twinge, pain and discharge and form a decision that it had or hadn't worked. And being told to 'relax' isn't helpful. Even now, at 29 weeks pregnant, the anxiety hasn't gone.

It also felt isolating and lonely, doing it all without the support of your friends and family, because you don't want to get anyone's hopes up unnecessarily or feel any extra pressure for it to be successful. I didn't want to talk about it with family as I knew they thought we should leave it, as we already have our first little boy.

It's also lost me a friendship with a good friend who was going through treatment at the same time. While ours was successful on the fifth try, hers didn't have the same happy ending we had both hoped for. Of course we had already imagined a future of doing baby classes together on maternity leave.

There is an understanding that stress is not helpful when trying to conceive, which makes things very tricky for parents who desperately want to have kids. How did you manage this?

I allowed myself to be sad and grieve. Jess was a huge support and tried to shield me from as much happy news from friends as he could, but I don't think he fully understood how I was feeling and at times it looked like I was jealous and bitter.

I bought myself an exercise bike, which was low impact, and did classes three times a week. Not only did it help me relax, but it made me feel great.

We went on holiday in between rounds when we could and made sure we still had plenty of family time, not letting the IVF process consume our lives and certainly not letting our little boy know about any of what was going on behind the scenes.

Thank you so much, Amanda, for sharing your story and your experience of stress around conception. It's a story that will help so many other people feel less alone.

Amanda's story reminds me how unhelpful it is – in any situation – to be told to relax. If someone is telling you to relax, it's either because they need you to or because they really don't fully under-stand your situation. Their advice may be well-meaning, but it often lands terribly. If we could all instantly chill out, we would, and I wouldn't have to write this book. If you find yourself the beneficiary of such advice, it is totally OK to state that you don't find it helpful or useful. If you experience intrusive questions, as Amanda did when trying to conceive, it is again completely OK to not answer or to say you would rather keep such matters private. Setting these sorts of boundaries is often imperative in keeping your own mental health in a good place.

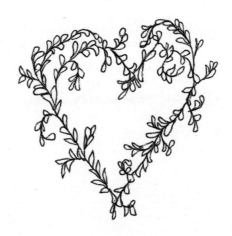

Little things to say when you are worried about a mate

If your friend is going through a stressful situation, it can be hard to know what to say. I have said the wrong things in the past and also acted awkwardly, struggling to find the right words of support. Here are some questions or statements you could use if you are navigating this with a friend or loved one.

❀ 'How can I be of help?'

❀ 'Do you feel supported?'

❀ 'I am here for you in whatever way you need.'

❀ 'Do you want to talk about it today, or would you rather we discuss something else?'

❀ 'I'm not going to try to fix you or the situation, but I see you, and I hear you.'

IT'S A SHAME

Looking back, the time I felt most out of control was when I was experiencing a huge bout of shame. I had been through some very tricky experiences that resulted in what I deem the ugliest of emotions. On its own, it feels almost impossible to navigate at the best of times, but lump stress on top of that and you're really spiralling. This might sound like a bold assumption, but I'm not sure you can feel shame without stress. For me, shame was a full-body experience. My own skin crawled with self-loathing. I felt suffocated, at times unable to even produce a squeak of a voice. The sound of my own vowels spoken aloud made me shudder. I wanted to hide, which in my job is almost impossible.

Pushing myself to leave the house each day felt stressful. Walking towards a row of flashing cameras outside Radio 1 made me want to burrow a hole in the pavement beneath me. Often, just seeing other humans felt stressful, as I feared they thought the same terrible thoughts about me that were whirring through my head.

I don't think there is a quick fix to ridding oneself of shame. In my experience it takes support, guidance and time. I have had intermittent therapy ever since this tricky patch and continue to explore techniques and practices that benefit my mental and physical health. If you are experiencing shame, the last thing you feel like doing is talking about it. But shame breeds in secrecy, so if you can talk to someone you will experience an instant shift. For starters, try writing a little about it below. This book cannot judge you. See how you feel once you've written down your thoughts.

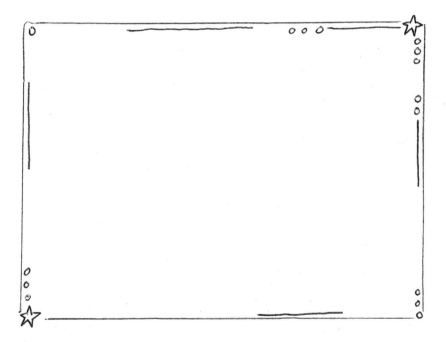

Read your words back and see if you would judge someone else as harshly as you judge yourself. I bet you wouldn't. Often, we pin shame to ourselves much more readily than we do to others.

Which areas of your life are affected by feelings of shame?

....

....

....

....

....

Little things to help reduce the stress of shame

❁ **Be patient with yourself.** Remember, it takes time to heal from periods of shame, so go gently and seek support from loyal friends or professionals who are willing to listen without judgement or hand out too much 'quick fix' advice.

❁ **Take little steps.** If you are feeling stressed about moving through this shame, think about your own limits and how much you're willing to push yourself. There is no rush or race with any of this. It's a long road that we are all on together. There is no winner or prize for getting there first.

✿ **Share your story.** Your words will undoubtedly be met with compassion and empathy, and you'll feel an instant relief in admitting your feelings to someone who cares about you. Your story might even be met with a similar one. I was once asked by a therapist to tell a story that brought me great shame. I stuttered my way through an excruciating anecdote, then sat in tension waiting for her to condemn me in some way. She then brilliantly told me a story that was steeped in shame for her. I laughed and told her that she had nothing to worry about. I didn't see her story as shameful whatsoever, and likewise she didn't see the shame in mine. A story shared is not only one halved, but one with a lot less shame and stress.

✿ **Talk to someone who won't judge you.** You may feel like there isn't a single person who would sit and listen to you without judgement, but I have an inkling there is. Everyone's had embarrassing moments or times of regret. If you still don't feel like there is someone who could help you, you could look into professional help. When you feel like the time is right, share your story, in order to dilute the shame and take back control.

❀ **Try to turn shame into embarrassment.** Notice that, as you start to work on your self-acceptance and lessen the stress around shame, some of the feelings may morph into embarrassment. Embarrassment is one level up from shame; it's like shame's slightly more amusing cousin. It may feel impossible to apply humour or levity to shame, but embarrassment allows you a little more freedom to reinterpret a situation.

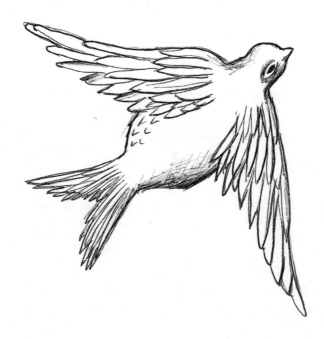

A little story on embarrassment, to help relieve your own ...

I once spent half of a podcast recording calling one of my guests the wrong name. It was on Zoom (which I find discombobulating), it was past 8pm, which is not my favoured time for cognitive brilliance, and I felt a strange panic set in just before. Looking back, I was overwhelmed and overtired, which is not a great recipe for success. Afterwards I fell into a pool of shame. I felt like the world's worst interviewer and a shitty person. This ate away at me for months, with shame nipping at my heels whenever the memory popped back into my mind to haunt me.

As time has passed, I can look at this situation with a little more distance and less heat. I have been called many an incorrect name over the years. Cab drivers have exclaimed to me that they're so excited to be driving Fern Britton around, and 'Oi, aren't you that bird off the telly?' is a familiar holler. Have I been offended? Not in the slightest. Will I hold a huge grudge forever? Not at all. If I'm able to be so forgiving of others, then why can't I forgive myself? With this in mind, the shame I felt at the time has been diluted with some self-kindness and now shows up as embarrassment. A healthy dose of embarrassment, that I can handle and sometimes even chuckle at.

Try it now. Is there a memory that sparks shame that you can transform into embarrassment? It doesn't have to morph into a hilarious anecdote, but the transition might take some of the stress away. Even writing down a shameful experience can lessen the heat. After you have written it here, sit up, look around and notice that the world is still spinning.

THE MESS I'M IN

When I feel the wheels spinning off and stress taking hold, I usually start making neat piles of belongings and straightening books on shelves. I need the visual of my surroundings to make sense and look ordered to help me cognitively catch up. When I was in the end stages of a relationship in my twenties, I found myself, one Saturday morning, on my knees, scrubbing brush in hand, frantically cleaning the stone tiles in the hallway. I wanted, perhaps needed, the floor to look spotless in order to cancel out the mess my life was in. At the time it seemed like the only action that could stop my entire world falling apart.

You may react to the feeling of being out of control in a comparable way, or perhaps you have the propensity to react in an opposing way. It's an interesting observation to make. Do you try to control the mess and stress by tidying, or do you create more mess to distract yourself from the stress you feel?

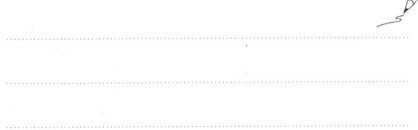

....

....

....

If you have found yourself obsessively cleaning to try and limit your own stress in these moments, could you view it as a nudge to look at what feels out of control in your life? Having that awareness is often a great starting point in making changes or lessening the pressure. If you find yourself drowning in mess, could you get curious about what you might be avoiding?

....

....

....

Spark joy

If you find yourself in visual mess and chaos at home, think about whether it makes you feel more stressed. If it does, could you have a small clear-out? Get rid of that yeti costume that you're keeping in case you get invited to a mythical creature fancy dress party. Chuck out the five extra spatulas you never use. Rid yourself of the vase in the cupboard your godmother got you that you don't actually like. Clearing space in your home gives you mental space. There are so many brilliant charity shops who will love you forever, too.

PHONES AND SCREENS

Say hello to the most obvious statement in this book, but it's one we all need to hear. Less time on screens equals less stress. We all know the ramifications of using our phones excessively, yet we still do it. I spend a lot of time on my phone and laptop working on Happy Place projects, but if I'm truly honest with myself, I could be a lot more disciplined about time off screen. Most of us feel like we don't have much control over how bombarded we are by the constant information we view on our screens, but we have a lot more of a say than we believe.

Melissa Urban, aka the Boundary Lady, who I've mentioned a few times already in this book, coined the term 'energy leakage', which refers to the amount of energy we lose by scrolling on social media, looking on news websites, texting people constantly and mindlessly browsing online. It's ever so normal to see full buses or trains of individuals glued to their phones, or people walking with their necks craned down to their screen. I'm often one of them. Each time we scroll on social media, or constantly chat in a WhatsApp group, we are expelling energy. We have an emotional reaction to everything we are seeing, reading and hearing, so without any breaks in this pattern, we are left depleted and drained. As well as the stress we might absorb from reading negative news stories or slipping into a game of comparison with others on Instagram, we are expelling energy while doing so.

On the other hand, if we're mindful of how we use our screens, we can of course feel boosted. Tech itself is benign: it's how we choose to use it that counts. Notice the moments where using technology is draining you. Do you feel boosted or drained from your screen time today?

....

If I have spent an inordinate amount of time scrolling, I feel like I've eaten a huge slice of very sugary, icing-laden cake. I'm as high as a kite, yet on the precipice of an energy plummet. The trough comes so quickly after the peak that the spike was barely there at all. How do you feel after you have been on your screen for too long?

....

....

NEGATIVE OVERLOAD

The older I get, the less capable I am of taking in any negative media. I do not have the energy for online arguments about what a Kardashian shouldn't have worn, violent or disturbing TV shows, edgy or aggressive messaging, or group WhatsApp chats that I can't keep up with. I know that if I am sucked into any of those areas I'll be left feeling on high alert, and that's not something I enjoy. These days I try to curate my intake of media to be positive, inspirational, and joyful. I follow individuals who discuss positive change and subjects I care about. I watch TV shows that leave me feeling boosted. I don't watch the news, which you may see as ignorant, but I would rather curate and search for global stories I can learn from and help with if possible. Make sure the media you are absorbing leaves you boosted and energised.

List below all the TV shows, podcasts, musical artists, books, websites, magazines and more that leave you feeling positive.

....

....

....

....

....

....

....

TIME AFTER TIME

The one aspect of life we have no control over is time. This can cause immense stress if we are stuck in the pain of the past or if we're obsessing about the future. The only way to combat this type of stress is by being present. Eckhart Tolle calls this being 'in the now'. Already today I have spent over 80 per cent of my time forward planning and thinking about how the rest of the day should pan out. If I'm not looking after myself, I also have the propensity to drift into the past and feel great stress about regrets I have. I have to remember I have no control over the past or future, so settling into the now is the only way to find some peace.

Little things to get you in the now

❀ **Focus on your breath and senses.** Sit for the next few minutes and just notice the sounds around you, the feel of your clothes, the smells and what you can see. Each time your mind wanders to a differing thought, just bring your aware- ness back to your breathing. Each time you manage to bring it back to your breath, your mind is in the present moment.

❀ **Know that you are safe in the present moment.** Unless you're actually running from a tiger, you can allow yourself to settle into the safety and peace of the now. You might say, 'But I can't, my life is a mess.' That mess is only your perceived mess of the past or your fear of things being a mess in the future. In this moment, there is no danger or threat. It's by no means an easy concept to weave into every second of the day, but when I manage to have little moments like this, things seem less stressful.

❀ **Challenge yourself to sit with discomfort.** If you feel discomfort in the now, know that your feelings cannot hurt you. If you're desperate for a glass of wine and feel yourself tensing up as you wish your day away, try sitting with the discomfort instead. I have to practise this daily, as I can easily be sucked into future worries about my kids, work or the big global issues. Rather than reaching for my phone to distract me, or eating a snack to numb the worry, I try to just sit with it. The unwelcome news is that it doesn't feel very nice. The good news is: it can't hurt you.

✻ **Remember: your stress cannot affect time.** Imagine you're in a car, driving to an important appointment, and the traffic becomes very heavy. In this moment you have two choices. You can slip into your habitual reaction, which might be to feel wildly out of control, feel your body tense up, shout at other drivers and grit your teeth. Or you can choose to accept that you might be late. Getting overly stressed out will not make time slow down or the traffic dissipate. We can choose to turn up flustered, adrenaline-fuelled and tense, or accepting and calm. It is of course much harder to do when there is more at risk, but the concept remains the same. Our stress cannot save us.

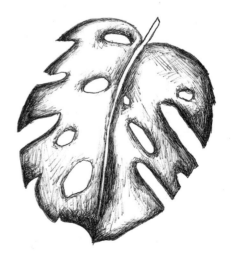

RELATIONSHIPS

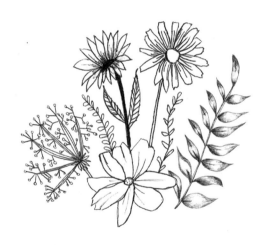

Relationships can offer support, comfort and safety, yet they can also be one of the biggest causes of stress. Some relationships are chosen by us, and some we find ourselves in without much say in the matter. We might cherish friendships that feed our soul, but also feel incredibly stressed by dealing with people that we find impossible. Reading Marc Schulz and Robert J. Waldinger's *The Good Life* opened my eyes to the direct correlation between healthy relationships and happiness. The message is clear: strong relationships create a good life. It's not our jobs, success, the perfect partner, fame, wealth or popularity that create it but simply our relationships with others.

Reading this book was the catalyst for a great shift in me. I'm often far too invested in my work life, as I attempt to reap happiness and self-worth via effort. After reading Marc and Robert's book, I started to see a successful day as one where I have properly connected with people. The other important lesson from the book is that the relationships that keep us happy, connected and less stressed don't have to be easy ones. You might fight with your partner, squabble with your best mate or find your neighbour challenging, but that shouldn't negate the worth of the relationship. If the balance tips and the relationship is bringing you more stress than comfort, that is where you have to make adjustments for your own sanity. This will require either setting boundaries or leaving the dynamic altogether. These situations are also another chance for us to look at how we are responding to stress and regain some control around the amount of stress we feel. In this section of the book, we'll look at how relationships can cause stress, but also how they can alleviate it and create space for peace and joy.

YOU CAN'T PICK THEM

As clichéd as that phrase can be, it is true. When it comes to families, we have no say over which one we're born into and the extended
members that will be along for the ride. Over my years of interviewing
people from all walks of life, hearing stories of fallouts and tension,
it seems that family issues are the most deeply rooted stresses of all.

Every single family has its troubles. There will always be those
family members who say too much or too little, who hold a grudge,
who take too much, behave inappropriately, and so on. They'll
be individuals that bring out the worst in you and dynamics so
well-trodden that you've forgotten there is room for change.

Which dynamic in your family causes you the most stress?

....

Why does it make you feel that way?

....

....

What is your current coping mechanism?

....

....

Do you believe it works?

....

....

Often, we create coping mechanisms to deal with a family situation the best we can under duress. Historically my own coping mechanism with an individual I find challenging has been to drop a text message hand-grenade into an already stressful situation. My rage has taken over and I haven't been able to sit in the discomfort and respond thoughtfully. This obviously leads to more stress, so I know that my coping mechanism does not work.

Little things to help when triggered by a relative

❀ **If you are usually quick to react when a family member stresses you out, try to say 'halt' in your head.** I like the word 'halt' as it sounds comedic and dramatic. Rather than counting to ten while attempting to breathe in a Zen-like way, just put the brakes on and hear a commanding voice in your head yell, 'HALT.' We all know that getting into a huge argument or reacting without thought is not going to work. By the way, I should point out that I sometimes still do this, in heated situations. I'm saying this for *me*, too. I am a fiery little arsehole some of the time, but again, I know reacting straight away from a place of stress doesn't work for me anymore.

❀ **Write a letter that you don't send.** Get a pen and go for it. Be as unfiltered as possible and release all the stress and pain you feel. Tell them why they are hurting you/disrespecting you/ irritating you and explain how that makes you feel. It can be as long or as short as needed. Then burn it. There is something beautifully ceremonial about burning a letter. You can turn it into a ritual, to set yourself free from the emotions in the dynamic. Go outside and make sure you are undisturbed. Then watch your letter burn and turn to ash. You might feel an instant lift from doing this, or perhaps a slow and incremental detachment from the situation. There is a whole section on ritual in my book *Bigger Than Us*, as I got to spend time with and learn from the amazing coach and medicine woman Alex Bedoya.

❄ **Record a voice note explaining how you feel.** Pretend you are talking to the other person. You can whisper, scream, shout, cry: there are no rules. But once you have recorded it, delete it. Getting the words out is incredibly cathartic, as it not only sets the words free but stops them getting stuck in your throat. When I experienced a large cyst on my vocal cords in 2019, I knew it was due to stuck words. Subsequently I always try to release them, so I don't end up with throat issues again.

If you feel you can speak to the other person in the dynamic in a truthful but measured way, think about how you might approach the situation. Could you meet in neutral territory? Could you send a text, outlining what you want to cover in your discussion, so you initiate the chat with some boundaries in place? Shaman Wendy Mandy taught me about the concept of talking sticks. This is a method used to enable healthy discussion. Whoever is holding the stick (it can literally be a stick, or hairbrush, or pen – anything) gets to talk. Rather than starting each statement with 'You make me feel/you did this', you begin by stating how you feel and taking ownership of your emotions. For example: 'I am struggling to find a way through this. I am feeling angry.' Once the talking stick has been passed over, the other person has the opportunity to speak without interruption. It might seem laborious or even ludicrous, but it hugely encourages true listening and keeps things from getting heated, as there is no talking over one another.

I've worked with a variety of healers and therapists over the years, and one practice I've often found insightful is a 'cutting of the cords' ceremony. If there is someone in your life who causes you great stress, but you're unable to leave the relationship, you can use this technique to create some emotional distance. You can also use this practice to release stress and tension from past dynamics that still cause you pain. It's a meditative practice, but you don't have to have meditated previously to do it. To begin, lie or sit down comfortably and close your eyes. Then imagine lots of different cords, running from your physical body to the other person's body. Think about where those cords are in your body. Do you feel them coming from your abdomen? Or your neck, or shoulders? Your head or feet? Think about what colour the cords are, what texture, what thickness. Once you have established how many cords there are and how they're connected to you, picture the other person sitting opposite you, with the other end of your cords attached to their physical body.

Notice all the areas of their body that connect to the cords. Then imagine a large pair of shining silver scissors in your hands. Hold them in front of you; notice how sharp the edges are. Then, when you are ready, cut each cord in your mind. See the ends of the cords drop to the ground and shrivel away. Cut each one until there are none left to cut.

It's a good idea to lie or sit in meditation for a few minutes after this ceremony, to process what you've worked on and to let the feelings percolate. You may notice an instant shift, or it may take a few days for you to notice that you feel lighter.

If you have experienced severe pain through lying, abuse or violence within your family, do seek professional help if you can, or access support groups or online forums. That kind of stress cannot be tackled by using this book alone.

PARENTING AND BLENDED FAMILIES

It is, of course, a joy and a privilege to bring up children, but it's also bloody stressful. Some days the responsibility of being a parent can feel overwhelming, and I had that realisation precisely two seconds after Rex was born. All my previous fantasies of becoming a chilled-out, kaftan-wearing, easygoing mum went out of the window the minute I held my gorgeous firstborn in my arms. Nothing can prepare you for that overwhelming sense of love, but also responsibility, heightened worry, and fear that you're getting it all wrong. Everyone tells you how the love and nurturing instinct is instant and urgent, but no one warns you about the instant stress. There seems to be a disproportionate amount of preparation for the labour itself and what one might pack in a cute overnight bag, or how many nappies you'll go through or what the best nipple cream is, yet there's truly little preparation for how you'll cope with the responsibility.

I've often asked myself whether it's possible to experience enormous amounts of love without stress. Can we dive into all-encompassing love without worrying about losing it? Parenting constantly teaches me that there can be two opposing emotions at play simultaneously; love and stress can sit side by side.

I am also acutely aware that all of us parents/carers will make mistakes. There is no way to be the perfect parent. All of those adverts or Instagram posts we see of kids dressed in matching, clean outfits, smiling at their calm and collected parents, represent 1 per cent of the truth. Of course there are beautiful moments of parenting: serene moments, miraculous moments, heart-pounding joy, but it's usually messy, noisy and painful too.

What do you find most stressful about parenting?

....

....

....

....

....

Little things we can do to reduce parenting stress

❀ **First up: we need to give ourselves a break.** Challenging the acerbic voice within that's telling us we are getting it wrong might seem impossible, but being aware it's there in the first place is a great start. We are often so used to an inner mono-logue that berates and self-flagellates that we forget it's not the truth. We start to believe our thoughts, which creates even more stress. If we can notice the ever-running commentary about how badly we are doing, then we can start to separate from it. We can challenge these negative ideas and work out how and when they were formed.

❀ **Look at what you are getting right.** Notice and celebrate all of the energy you've put into parenting. Applaud yourself for getting out of bed at 6am on a Saturday. Pat yourself on the back for remembering to pack the school snack. I so often forget to take note of what I *am* doing as I'm so focused on what I'm *not* doing.

❀ **Stop comparing yourself and your kids to other people.** There are countless times I've witnessed someone else's kid chow down on a huge stem of broccoli while mine get up from the table announcing they want cereal, and then fallen into a spiral of compare and despair. I've looked at other families and worried that I'm not putting enough effort in with the kids' reading or homework and have panicked when other kids could swim properly while mine were still in armbands. I have the propensity to blame myself for everything, so I've often used all this information as ammunition against myself. I have learned and am still learning that it doesn't help anyone to compare yourself to others. Every child develops at a different rate and everyone parents differently. All we can do is our best and seek peace in that.

❀ **Work out what your values are and stick to them.** This point follows on from my previous one, as we can only find peace in our methods and decisions if we truly believe in them. If we feel placing importance on eating well is a priority, then we might not worry so much that our children aren't potty trained at the same time as everyone else's. If we know that music is important to us, we can worry less that our kids aren't nailing maths. If manners are top of the list, then it might not be such a big deal that our kids hate after-school clubs. Know your values and work to them instead of reaching for perfection in all areas.

❀ **Seek comfort and connection.** Share your worries with friends who might have similar stories to tell. There is nothing better than hearing someone else's parenting struggles or mishaps. I will treacherously admit that I love seeing other people's kids kick off in the supermarket, as it makes me feel less alone in the mess of parenting. I feel no irritation or judgement towards them at all. In those moments, my heart floods with empathy and total relief that someone else is going through it too.

❀ **Don't feel guilty for taking time for yourself.** I have exclusively written that sentence for me. I am a guilt harvester, so I find it exceedingly difficult to allow myself time out without drowning in guilt. A great parent/carer is not one who is available 24/7 without a break. We all need time out with friends, or in solitude, to rest, recuperate, laugh and remember who we are.

Blended

I met my husband when my stepchildren were five and nine. I went from being a 29-year-old single woman to having two small kids running around the house. I feel lucky that my experience of step-parenting has been positive but, like in any family dynamic, there are challenges and stressful moments to shoulder too. Navigating blending two families, taking on children that aren't biologically yours, or having your kids enter another household can be challenging. There will be compromise, difficult conversations, less free time or perhaps more time alone if your kids are going to your ex-partner's, a lack of control and new boundaries to set. I blindly walked into step-parenting without much thought about how my life would change. I learned on the job and at times felt alone in the discombobulation of my new life.

Little things to help navigate a blended family

❀ **Reach out to others who may be going through something similar.** I was fortunate enough to have a good friend navigating her relationship with a new partner's kids around the same time, so we've often acted as a sounding board to one another in times of confusion or stress.

❀ **Keep up a good line of communication with your partner from the start.** If you are taking on their kids, or vice versa, make sure you constantly talk about what works and what doesn't and understand that you'll often be coming from quite different angles on certain matters. You don't have to agree on everything, but compromise has to be reached to create more peace for you and the kids.

❀ **Include the kids in as many decisions as possible.** If you are planning a holiday, or redecorating part of the house, include the children so they don't feel out of the loop. When Jesse and I got married, Arthur and Lola chose the flavours of each tier of our wedding cake. We wanted them to feel a part of the day, rather than participants who had little say in the matter. We've included Arthur and Lola in as many decisions as possible, especially in the early days when they were experiencing a lot of change too.

❀ **Know that it's OK to make mistakes and feel stressed out.** Blending a family takes a lot of work, effort and mental flexibility. So go easy on yourself and know you're doing your best.

❀ **Drop the guilt.** If you feel guilty for taking time for yourself, getting things wrong, or for feeling resentful, try to park the guilt. Taking time out is essential for balance: everyone makes mistakes, and having emotions is not a criminal offence. If you feel angry or resentful, just sit with it. You don't have to feel guilty for being an imperfect parent or step-parent. Have your feelings, notice them, allow them to be there, then maybe write them down or talk to someone about them. There's nothing wrong with feeling emotions, but we do need to have self-awareness so our actions are not informed by them. Feel anger, but don't pass it onto someone undeserving. Feel resentment, but don't throw it in someone else's face. Feel the annoyance, but don't take it out on another. Feel it, own it, but don't pass it on.

Check out Kate Ferdinand's brilliant podcast, *Blended*, to hear from other people going through the same things. She has also written an incredibly insightful book called *How To Build A Family*, which is packed with anecdotes and professional advice.

Teenage kicks

If you have a teenager in your life, you will know what a bumpy time it can be. Hormones are flying, priorities are changing, peer groups are influencing, and bodies are transforming, as these once tiny people try to bridge the gap between childhood and adulthood. As a parent or carer, you may feel completely unable to handle the challenges of the teen years. You might also be pushed away by your teen, who doesn't want your advice or help.

A friend of mine who now has older children once said to me that it's OK to just plod alongside your teenager, even if they are pushing you away. You don't have to try to fix them or challenge them too much; plodding alongside them will let them know you're there and will help lessen the stress of the rejection you might feel. Once my friend's teenager reached his twenties, they established a new phase and get along very well. The teen years do not last forever. I will say, though, that if you have an angelic teenager who causes you no stress at all: lovely stuff, carry on as you were.

If your teenager is experiencing something a little more severe than the average teen behaviour, do seek professional help. If they are self-harming, experiencing eating disorders, using alcohol or drugs or involved in any kind of crime, these challenges are often too big to deal with on your own.

Children with disabilities

Many studies show that parents of children with a disability or disabilities have the most prolonged experience of stress. Often the daily challenges are physically and mentally demanding, the practicalities of doctors' appointments or operations stressful, and the worry about future health extremely taxing. Over-tiredness and a lack of support can lead to emotions such as frustration, anger and maybe even shame, all of which increase stress. With a lack of government-led support, families are often forced to raise funds via charities or personal endeavours to cover the costs of equipment needed or house refurbishments that meet the child's needs.

Interview with my friend Abbie

Abbie, tell us about your beautiful family.

A: So in our family there's me and my husband Rich, my daughter Bea, and my and Rich's twins Ted and Monty. Plus Willow the dog and Rosie the cat.

Bea is 15 and very sensible! I do pinch myself over this, as I was definitely NOT the same as a teenager. Then there are Ted and Monty, who are eight years old. Ted is two minutes older than Monty and they are identical twins. They were born at 36 weeks during a planned C-section, which you are advised to have with identical twins. Both came out weighing exactly 5lbs 1oz each and they both had identical measurements, so they really were the same in every way, except that as they started to grow bigger we noticed Ted's head wasn't growing at the same rate as Monty's. He also had terrible acid reflux; if any parent has come across this in their children, it is just awful. He would scream continuously, day and night, to the point where one neighbour who lived next door (who we didn't know very well) commented on how patient I was with him.

A few months went by, with terrible feeding issues and Ted's head still not growing properly and looking flat at the back. We were told it was a twin thing as they had been so squashed inside of me. By eight months we decided to go to a private hospital, as we knew deep down something wasn't right and we just needed answers. We had various scans and tests and were given the news that no parent ever wants to hear, which is that Ted had suffered hypoxia just before my C-section and it was going to have a significant effect on his life. Basically, Ted was starved of oxygen and had extensive brain damage. Ted was diagnosed with 4-limb cerebral palsy, epilepsy, microcephaly (small head, where his brain damage has affected his head growth), laryngomalacia (a floppy larynx associated with cerebral palsy) and he is severely visually impaired. Ted is non-verbal and is immobile. He can't do anything for himself and we are his full-time carers. However, Ted lights up a room and is a master at getting what he wants from people. He has the most infectious giggle. Monty is kind and caring and sees the good in everyone. All my children are my everyday heroes.

There are so many studies that now show parents of kids with a disability have the most prolonged stress. Can you talk to me about the daily and long-term stresses you face?

The biggest stress for us as a family, especially for myself, is to recognise that you are living in a completely different world to the majority of other families, who have neurotypical children, and to not compare ourselves to them. It is very difficult, because for Ted's siblings you are trying to keep life as 'normal' as possible (whatever normal is) but the reality is that our lives are completely different. We can't sit down and put on a movie for us all to enjoy because Ted can't see it or understand it. We try to play a board game, but one of us has to hold and entertain Ted by singing or bouncing, while trying to roll a dice and be engaged with the other kids. Going out for family meals is tricky as Ted has a pureed food diet, so it takes a lot of planning and organising. If Ted decides he doesn't like the acoustics in a restaurant or a museum then it's game over and we have to leave, so trampolining, ice skating or anything that involves an activity are really hard now that he's so much bigger.

Then there are the hospital appointments. No two weeks are the same: there are appointments in various hospitals and clinics for Ted's treatments and we're constantly seeing different specialists and physicians with regard to his condition. We could be at one hospital one day for his epilepsy management and then across London to another hospital to manage his muscle tone. Then there are regular appointments to measure his reflexes, and ones to check his spine and hips due to his being non-weight-bearing. Some appointments will inevitably lead to another conversation about a condition we were unaware of, and then as result of that there will be a different specialist we have to see. It's an ever-evolving situation.

I view it very much like a boat moving down the river, stopping off from time to time to pick up passengers and drop them off, but the river never comes to an end. Long-term stress very much arises from the unknown: we don't really know where we will end up or ultimately how it will end for Ted. We know that eventually Ted's condition will mean that he probably won't have the same life expectancy as Monty, for example. I try not to go there in my head; I am, and have to be, very much in the present.

There is clearly not enough support for parents like yourself. What would be helpful, in terms of your own stress management and support network?

Recognising that the stress we are under on a continual basis takes its toll. It's not as though there's an end date and you are working towards that goal. It's continuous and constantly moving and evolving. I feel that parents like myself should be offered professional help in the form of therapy or counselling. I have a good network of mums in the same situation as myself, but no two children are the same, even if they have the same diagnosis. What works for some families doesn't necessarily work for others. There are days when I feel I just need to talk to someone who's going to understand what I'm faced with, with no judgement.

How do you cope with the stress you face?

Knowing that it may be unbearable now but this feeling won't last forever is one of my coping mechanisms. There was a time, a year or so ago, where Ted ended up going into A&E

with a strange breathing pattern. At first I just thought, 'It's Ted, there's always something new and unusual; it'll be fine.' Then the doctors started talking about being referred to a specialist hospital and that his oxygen levels were being affected. All of a sudden I found myself back in the place where we first had Ted's diagnosis; all noise drifted away and I felt like a stranger, looking into the unknown.

In those moments, I take a deep breath and tell myself, 'I can do this – I HAVE to do this, I don't have a choice.' I remember my dad giving me a card once that read: 'It's going to be all right in the end. If it's not all right, it's not the end.' Although it may seem an odd thing to say, given my situation, I very much try to live in the present, not the past and not the future. Tomorrow is always a new day, with new experiences. I don't want to one day wake up and feel regret that I wished that time in my life away, because even on those days, Ted has it so much harder than me and I want to make as many memories as I can, even the ones that are tough on the soul.

I also try to compartmentalise my stress, for example, I try not to not sweat the small stuff, like worrying about work, or friendship groups, or a five-hour flight delay, or my house flooding. None of those situations are ideal, but in the grand scheme of things they're not the end of the world. Letting go of my worries and not thinking miles into the future is a big weight off my shoulders – I feel happier because of it.

How does the stress show up physically for you?

Exhaustion. EXHAUSTION! We get very little sleep with Ted; he can sometimes wake up only once in the night, but other times he can be up for hours. I've made changes to my life-style to allow for the constant exhaustion. I eat really well (even if it's just snacks, because I don't always have time to sit down for a meal), with lots of vitamins and supple-ments. I don't drink; I take our dog Willow out most days for a two-hour walk if I can. I need that time to reflect and reset. I don't give myself a hard time because I can't exercise as much as I want to, or meet my mates for drinks, or have any social life to speak of. I power nap wherever I can, even if it's just ten minutes before the school run. I know that one day I may just run out of steam, but in the meantime I'm giving myself every chance I can to make it to the end.

Abi's strength, resilience and coping mechanisms have inspired me and helped me so much over the years. My biggest takeaway is for us not to beat ourselves up when we don't have time for taking care of ourselves. We hear about the benefits of self-care a hell of a lot but what about when there is simply no time? What we don't need in times of stress is to then beat ourselves up that we are not perfecting self-care. That totally defeats the object. On days where time is tight and responsibilities are huge, self-care can simply be practised as refusing to beat yourself up that you're not doing traditional self-care.

Abi, you are simply amazing. Thank you for sharing your story.

Helping neurodiverse children

If your child has been diagnosed with ADHD, OCD, ASD, dyslexia, dyspraxia or any other neurodivergent condition, then you will also find yourself with the stress of managing their needs and behavioural traits. Even obtaining a diagnosis can be stressful. I'm very interested in progressing my understanding of neurodivergent brains, as there are some in my family and close circle. I recently completed a month-long online course to learn more, which was eye-opening.

There are varying presentations of these diagnoses, and everyone will, of course, exhibit them differently. Getting to know how your, or your child's, brain works can be incredibly relieving, so if you have ever wondered if your struggles, or gifts in life, stem from being neurodivergent you might want to explore seeking professional help in getting a diagnosis.

If you have a diagnosis already it's important that you and your child focus on the gifts that the diagnosis provides, rather than just the challenges ahead. For example, some gifts could be hyperfocus in certain areas, innovative thinking, creativity or strong character traits that have helped you or could help your child later in life.

If you or your child is neurodivergent, write a little about the positives this diagnosis brings.

....

....

....

....

....

Your family set-up

The western world has focused all its attention on the nuclear family set-up. Gone are the days of the village mentality, where neighbours, grandparents, aunties and uncles would raise kids collectively. I'm not sure how we begin to move back to a society that holds those values, as we have years of unpicking to do. Yet knowing our stress is valid is a good starting point. When we are stressed and feel we can't cope, it's usually because we believe we *should* be able to cope. But if we look at how little support we have in raising our children, is it really any surprise so many of us are so stressed out?

If you feel stressed out and guilty when it comes to juggling work and family life, the number one thing that helps me is to be kinder to myself. Self-compassion has the ability to dilute guilt and stress, but we have to get into the habit of it. Each day, remind yourself that you are juggling a lot and that it's OK to feel stress. Tell yourself you are doing your best and that is enough. Form a new daily habit that allows you to focus on how well you are doing under the circumstances, rather than how much you're *not* doing.

Stress is a totally reasonable reaction to what you're experiencing, but when stress feels relentless, you may need to make changes. If the daily stress of juggling work and family life is taking a mental or physical toll on you, change is needed. Can you reach out and ask for help? Don't feel like a failure for asking for help: it's often essential. Is there anyone who can take your child to school for you? Could a willing neighbour pick up some extra bits on the weekly food shop? Might someone at work help unburden your load? Even when we feel there is no help available, there often is. We just forget to ask. At times I have felt I can't ask, because I should be coping with everything on my own. No one is going to give me a medal for doing it all and often people are more than happy to help, as it gives them a boost to know that they're helping. Ask for help. You deserve it.

I need space

Finding space is the part of parenting I find most challenging. Sometimes it feels like the walls are closing in and I can't move for questions, mess and noise. I often prioritise family and work and put myself at the bottom of the pile. My martyr tendencies highlight the fact that inside, I don't believe I deserve any time out at all.

The guilt drives me to overachieve at work and to give every other moment to my kids. Subsequently I end up feeling burned out and even more stressed. I'm actively trying to right my tendencies to put everyone before myself, but it certainly doesn't come naturally.

little things

I think many women feel the same. On the opposite page, write a list of responsibilities in your life and see where you fit into that list. Are you at the top or way down at the bottom of the pile?

You don't have to fill out the whole list. Your list can be as long or short as you need. The amount is irrelevant; the position of where you fit into it all is what counts.

Can you move yourself up at least one spot on that list this week? Remember the old saying: you have to put your oxygen mask on before you attend to anyone else. I am saying this for me as much as for you, as I'm currently quite far down the old list.

MY PRIORITIES

1 ....

2 ....

3 ....

4 ....

5 ....

6 ....

7 ....

8 ....

BREAK-UPS AND BREAKDOWNS

One of the most stressful relationship dynamics is a break-up. Whether married or not, choosing not to be with someone, or being on the receiving end of that decision, is incredibly tough. Alongside sorrow, discombobulation, heartache, and the practical issues of a break-up is stress. Even if you wanted out of the relationship and actively moved towards it, you will experience stress alongside the liberation.

This flavour of stress can be found in all corners of the day. In conversation with colleagues, who quiz you about your partner; when boxing up belongings that need to be moved out; when cancelling holidays that had been booked for two. Those initial months are a trudge through stress and sorrow. The practical side of it is almost as taxing as the mental exhaustion. You may even experience physical symptoms from the stress, like backache, headaches or an irritable digestive system. All of this is normal. Let's hear from a friend of mine: entrepreneur, business founder and mother to my godson Bram, Liz MacCuish.

Interview with Liz

Liz, divorce is listed as one of the most stressful things a person can go through. Can you tell us a little about your divorce and how it affected you?

LM: I would wholeheartedly agree with that statement. Every divorce is different, so even if friends have gone through one before you, it's really hard to give any helpful advice. Also, I was the first of my friends to go through this, so it was very much learning by doing. Del and I met in 2004 and I was pregnant within six months. It really fast-tracked everything because, though it was a new relationship, as soon as I found out I was expecting, I was sure I wanted to be a mum. Bram was born, prematurely, in September 2005 and spent his first few months in special care. A really intense time for us all. My and Del's relationship definitely had a few wobbles in those early months, but we were both really committed parents. My work schedule was also really demanding, and I travelled frequently. In 2009 I gave birth to my second son, Gabe. In 2012 I had my twins, Teddy and

Wren, and life became the true definition of hectic. Four kids and running a growing business. Something had to give, and ultimately it was our marriage.

A chance trip away with a girlfriend in April 2015 was just the space I had been craving, to be with myself, my thoughts. On the penultimate day, somewhere up a mountain in the Ibizan hills, I suddenly felt the clarity I didn't even realise I had been longing for. I wanted out, but how? How would it work in real terms, financially, and how would we tell the kids?

The one thing I knew – because I think, in most cases you do really know – was that Del felt the same way. But I also knew it would take me to start the conversation. I came home from that trip and we had a really healthy and expansive chat, tons of tears, but we were calm. We agreed we both wanted out and then, over the days and weeks that followed, the enormity of the decision hit us both, in huge ugly waves of guilt, fear and resentment. All the emotions. In my job I'm used to finding solutions, to creating impactful and creative strategies, so I used that same ingenuity to make a very practical plan to end our marriage, in the least painful way possible.

I will say, those months were just awful. I confided in a few close friends and my mum, but we couldn't really tell anyone else, and it was like keeping an awful secret. My eyes were so puffy I looked like I had some awful allergic reaction (which was what I went with if anyone asked). I can't tell you how strange it is to make a life-changing decision like that, but to still share a bed with that person. I would heartily recommend anyone reading this finds an alternative option, even if it's the sofa. You need your own space. Any intimacy feels like going in the wrong direction. I wrote and rehearsed a script for weeks, to tell the kids why their parents had decided to split. But in the end, I couldn't remember any of it. I just remember sitting the older two down on the sofa (the twins were too young) and explaining that they were our priority, but that we couldn't commit to being together as parents any more. I think there was only ever going to be one outcome. They were so angry and upset. A piece of that day will stay with me forever, like a paper cut. But, like with so many things, time does heal somewhat.

The next few weeks were a blur, but thankfully we had a trip to France booked and I took the kids on my own for a week with friends. It was just the tonic we all needed, and we didn't have to be brave, we just had to *be*, because we were with our best friends.

The next year was hard. Really hard. Though Del and I had been distant for years leading up to the split, I had never felt loneliness like it. I had plenty to keep me occupied during the day, but the evenings were brutal. I drank too much, and wallowed. If I had my time again, I would have taken a much more healthy path to healing. That year was relentless; the kids and work were all-consuming, and there was no time for me. At some point, spurred on by not wanting to end up alone with no one to share my life with, I started to look for little steps to rebuild. I took up Pilates and loved it. I spent more time in nature, ate better, got stronger, more resourceful, and we started to discuss divorce. We both agreed it would be amicable, but I definitely took control.

I knew we didn't have money for expensive lawyers, and we were amicable enough to use a mediator. I would recommend this route to anyone who feels they can use it. It's a one-off cost, and so much more straightforward than using a divorce lawyer. We saved tens of thousands of pounds.

I'm now five years into the most nourishing, rewarding and equal relationship with my new husband, Al, and I want to share that there are second chances there, for all of us to take. We just have to be strong and brave enough to take them.

I'm 48 this year, and in many ways, and largely thanks to Al and his magical reframing ways, I'm choosing to see this chapter as a rebirth.

I'm just getting started. On me.

What helped ease the stress?

Time. In all honesty. Talking to good friends, being kind to myself and taking care of myself.

Did you talk to others who could help or understand during the process?

In the first year I was definitely more withdrawn. Every day felt like climbing a mountain and I would crawl into bed, exhausted and teary, having anxiety about the next, repetitive day ahead. I shut people out and pretended I was OK more than I should have. I felt shame when I needn't have. I should have accepted more help. You really learn who loves you in those months.

You are now remarried and extremely happy, but blending a family can also be very stressful. How did you navigate this?

When Al and I made the decision to introduce each other to our kids, we had enjoyed a first-class romance for six months. Privately. I wanted to be sure that the person I introduced to my kids to was going to stick around. I met Al's son Buddy first, when he was eight. We had lunch and hit it off immediately. It felt like a relief to know we could bond. I was myself and didn't try too hard. I think that's key – kids can sniff out an over-trier a mile off! Next, I introduced Al to my kids, but we broke it up a bit as I thought it might be too much, all round, to do all four at once! Al came to meet the twins and we took them to the theatre. It went brilliantly. He then met the boys, and again, it went well. The next, far more daunting, step was to bring Buddy into our tribe. An only child, meeting four siblings! My son Gabe and Al's son Buddy are the same age, though very different, so we decided to introduce the boys to each other, on their own, first.

From day one they have got on brilliantly and this, my friends, is pure luck. We created the space, but we could not have conjured up the chemistry. We are so, so fortunate. In many ways, their relationship now, five years on, is our greatest achievement as a family.

The kids are all at different stages and we have three teens now, which of course brings all sorts of challenges, but we face them together as a team and it feels like a much more rewarding parenting experience. In fact, I no longer say I have four kids – I always say five, and so does Al. It feels right to say that.

What kind of relationship do you have with stress? How do you tend to react in a stressful situation?

I tend to tackle stress head on, in the moment. I try not to bury it. Doing the task you dread first is something I have carried into my everyday. It's a steadfast way to avoid procrastination, which normally prolongs my stress.

The squad

If you are going through a break-up or divorce it is important to create your own support squad around you. They don't have to know each other or even be in your life. Let me explain. I once heard from a woman who had a sick husband that she created her own imaginary support squad using people she admired. The list included incredible women like Debbie Harry, Tori Amos and Kate Bush. She would imagine them sitting around her husband's hospital bed and would ask them to pray with her.

Your support squad can consist of real friends and people you simply admire. Maybe pick a friend you know you can cry with, a relative you can vent to, a work colleague you can laugh with, an icon you can bring along for imagined support.

Write down your dream support squad below. What do you need and from who? Imagined or real, go for it.

....

....

....

....

New partnerships

Reading Jay Shetty's book *8 Rules of Love* opened my eyes to the stages of falling in love. Starting new relationships had always felt very chaotic to me. Love, lust and excitement would usually override common sense. Jay's explanation seemed neater, more organised and a lot less stressful. He suggests approaching new relationships with curiosity, communication and at a slower pace. I have always been urgent and have a tendency to rush things. Moving at a slower, more considered pace reduces stress when meeting new people.

How do you approach dating?

....

....

....

....

....

....

If, like me, you tend to rush into a new relationship, get curious about why. I know that alongside excitement at the start of a relationship runs fear, a fear that things won't work out. It's as if I rushed into new relationships to get as much as I could out of them in case they ended. This obviously isn't the healthiest approach. A much less stressful route to a new relationship is to take things slowly. Retrospectively, I can see that if I had been a little more curious about the fear I felt, I could have done something to address my own insecurities.

Don't rush: be curious about the feelings that arise for you, and know you deserve love.

Little things to help reduce the stress of dating

✿ **Turn up as you.** You are brilliant and enough as you are. In the past I often tried to be more pleasing to men by morphing into a 'better' version of myself in the hope they would like me, and it never ends well. Just be you. When I was about to go on the first date with my now husband, I got some stellar advice from Richard Curtis. If you're going to get romantic advice from anyone, let it be the man responsible for *Four Weddings and* a *Funeral*. I was stressing about what to wear and he asked me what I was wearing when Jesse had asked me on the date. I told him it was a skirt and a George Michael T-shirt. He said, 'Wear that then. It's an outfit you would wear normally, so just be you.' I worried the outfit was too casual, but took his advice and wore it on date one, and well, the rest is history. Thank you, Richard.

❀ **Don't bring your history to the table.** If you have been dumped or hurt in the past, remember this is a new situation unrelated to those times. Try to turn up with a clean slate.

❀ **Don't overthink it.** If you feel stressed about potential rejection, remember that if they're not right for you, they're not right for you. I have taken rejection very personally in the past but it's not a reflection of who you are or of your worth.

❀ **Take things slowly.** As in my aforementioned admission, I have never done this. Not once have I allowed a relationship to naturally, slowly unfurl. I have charged forward with urgency and no doubt missed vital opportunities to set necessary boundaries. Take Jay Shetty's advice and progress things at a snail's pace.

THE LONG ROAD

Being in a long-term relationship may offer support and a shoulder to lean on in stressful times, but that doesn't mean they are always easy. I have been with my husband Jesse for 12 years and have realised that any long partnership takes effort and work. You may encounter many an image of lovers holding hands, in complementary outfits, staring into each other's starry eyes and wonder what the hell you are doing wrong. Love underpins my marriage, but communication, empathy and a willingness to compromise are all vital in keeping our relationship healthy, and these are all things you don't see in an Instagram post. We've also never worn complementary outfits. Choosing effort and constant communication might not be the sexiest option, but I have learned it is essential to navigate a long-term relationship.

You may find that the more years you have under your belt in your relationship, the more you notice how different you and your partner are. Their way of doing things may differ from yours and this may cause you stress, but it's important that you communicate despite the differences. The reasons you're different from your partner should create interesting conversation and balance. If you notice the stressful times have started to outweigh the happier times, you may need to make changes. Stress is normal in a long relationship, but high levels of daily stress are not good for either of you, or your physical health and long-term happiness.

How stressful is your partnership?

....

Do you believe it is worth the stress?

....

Is the stress disproportionately more prominent than the love?

....

How could you set new boundaries, or start a conversation for positive change with your partner, to reduce stress?

....

....

....

FRIENDSHIPS

The end of a friendship can be equally as painful as the end of a romantic relationship, and it can often be much more confusing. A friendship rarely ends with belongings packed into a box, or the words 'it's over'. There is no agreement that you will move on, be seen with other people and permanently extracted from the other person's story. These things are all exclusively saved for romantic closure, and because there is rarely a clear ending, we often feel strange about grieving. If it's a friend who is woven through decades of your life it can be heartbreaking. If it's one of very few friends you have in your life, it can leave you feeling extremely lonely. If it's some-one you believe you have given a lot to, it can be deeply confusing.

From experience I believe there are two types of friendship break-up. The 'instant implosion', or 'the fade'. The instant implosion ends with a bang. A big argument or seminal moment in your friendship leaves you both wondering why you were friends in the first place. Angry words are spoken, and the foundations of your friendship rocked irrevocably. This kind of ending is stressful in the moment for most, as our defences go up and we feel the pain of years of friendship corroding, yet that stress can live on. I had a friendship end in this way a while back and every now and then this person enters my head. In these moments, an instant ball of stress lands heavily in my chest. I wonder how I could have done things differently. I question whether changing my approach could have saved the friendship, or if the other person involved had felt it was too late anyway. I've pondered whether I should approach them to see if we could work together to rebuild our friendship, but something tells me the timing isn't quite right. Maybe it's wrong to waste time waiting for the 'right' moment, but then again maybe this friendship was always going to fizzle out over time. There is no rule that you have to maintain all of your friendships: sometimes people come into your life for a certain amount of time and then exit.

Have you had a friendship end in a similarly stressful way? If so, write a little bit about how it ended below.

....

....

....

....

Do you believe recovering this friendship would cause more stress or less?

....

....

....

If you believe that attempting to rekindle this friendship would bring more stress, it might be best to leave things as they are for now. When I find myself worrying about my own friendship that ended this way (usually at 3am), I remember good times I spent with this person in the past and try to compartmentalise the pain of our break-up. I attempt to do so without guilt, shame or heartache. I just give thanks for what we once had and box those memories up. I don't want to tarnish the better times with how things have turned out. Then I send that person love.

You can practise this in meditation. It might feel impossible at first, so only practise this when you are ready. Close your eyes and picture the friend in question. Detach from the stories you've created about them: the pain, the angry words thrown your way, the differences of belief. Just picture them and then imagine sending a beam of white light their way. Sit in meditation and imagine sending them love via this beam of light for as long as feels right to you. If this person has badly hurt you, then you might start off attempting this for only a couple of minutes. You can build up over time. You might not believe they deserve your love, but this is to release you from the stress. If you can send them love yet simultaneously accept that your friendship has expired it will offer you peace and release tension.

I was once hurt by someone, and the pain plagued me for months. I had read about this concept of sending tricky people love in the book *Feel the Fear and Do It Anyway* by Susan Jeffers, and instantly thought: 'I can't do that.' Because the thought scared me so much, I knew I needed to do it. I was on holiday at the time so swam out into the sea, lay on my back, and imagined their face. I sent them love for maybe five seconds before I quit. The next day I did the same for a few more seconds, and the next day even longer. After practising this for many weeks I started to feel a lightness in my bones. When I pictured their face, I felt neutral. No pain, or resentment or anger. It didn't lead to an instigation of friendship repair, but it helped me feel a lot less stressed about it.

The fade

As well as the explosive endings to friendships, there are also the ones that slowly fade without reason or a noticeable turning point where things turned sour. There may be a less potent flavour of stress with this sort of friendship expiration, but we can still be left with big questions and concerns. If a friendship has slowly faded away in your life, can you see why? Is there a geographical distance between you, differing values or priorities, or a change in either of your lives? Write a little about it below.

....

....

....

Are you happy with how the friendship has drifted? Or would you feel happier if it was back on track? What steps could you take to heal this friendship?

....

....

Toxic people

We can find ourselves embroiled in friendships that cause nothing but pain. I'm sure we can all think back to dynamics in our life where the balance was off. Times where we were used as a verbal punchbag, a dumping ground, or undervalued. The friendship may have formed on good terms, or a casual basis due to circumstances, then taken a turn for the worse over time. Changes in friendship dynamics are often incremental, so they can be hard to spot at first. It's only later down the line that we wonder how we ended up in a toxic dynamic and how the hell we can get out of it.

In my forties, I really don't want friendships that stress me out. Life is too short, and I've realised that less is more. I have a handful of strong friendships that bring me nothing but joy and I am much less stressed out.

Are you in a toxic friendship?

YES   NO

If yes, how do you feel after spending time with this person?

....

What is keeping you in the friendship?

....

Would you feel less stressed out without this person in your life?

....

Little things to help reduce stress in friendships

❀ **Less is more.** Spend time with people who float your boat and boost your bounty. Courageously let go of toxic people.

❀ **Try healing the rift.** Move towards friendship repair if you are desperately missing someone who has faded from your life. Sometimes the second time round things are even better.

❀ **Don't stay in friendships for history's sake.** A friendship can be built on the past to a degree but it's not a strong enough foundation for a stress-free bond.

❀ **Make decisions that keep your mental health balanced.** Healthy debate is a beautiful part of being friends with some-one, but not if it turns into regular conflict.

LONELINESS

If you live on your own out of choice or otherwise, or are in a relationship that does not serve you, you might experience loneliness and feel you have to shoulder your stress on your own. Carrying the complexities of life without someone to talk to, to help process thoughts, can be tough. Sadly, due to our excessive use of technology, the fact that more of us move away from where we grew up for our jobs, and with the speed at which we live, more people feel lonely than ever before. We are connected by devices and the digital world, but true human connection, eye contact, and human touch are on the downward slide. As much as I love the community and conversation of the online world and social media, in-person human connection cannot be rivalled. If you feel you are lacking this in your own life, where could you find it? Is there a local activity or initiative you could be involved with? Perhaps a neighbour you could talk to for the first time? Or an old friend you miss and want to reconnect with? Who could you start up a conversation with today?

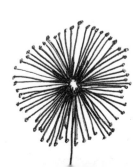

SPARKS OF CONNECTION

Over the next week, come back to this page and write down any small moments of meaningful connection. They don't have to be huge moments. Just little sparks of connection. Eye contact with the cashier in your local shop; smiling at a neighbour. It all counts and helps reduce the stress of feeling lonely.

1 ....

2 ....

3 ....

4 ....

5 ....

6 ....

7 ....

8 ....

PUBLIC-FACING ROLES

You might not think of working dynamics with strangers as relationships, but they are micro-moments that can either boost us or tip us over the edge when it comes to stress. Whilst researching stress, I spoke to individuals who work in customer service and public-facing roles. Having to calmly deal with people who are disgruntled, annoyed and urgent can be highly stressful.

One of my oldest mates, Fran, is an air steward, and she told me about the stress of putting on a smile on bad days, even for the rudest passengers. Fran deals with the stress by remembering she will not see these people again. This helps reduce the pressure she often feels. If she is yelled at or someone is rude to her, she limits her stress by remembering that the working day will have an end, unlike some stresses outside of work that do not. Fran also explained that in her role, you are often victim to tired passengers who are simply having a dreadful day. Over the years she has learned that not everybody is flying off on holiday. She has spoken to passengers over the years that are flying home for funerals and other challenging life events. She always tries to remember that you never know someone's full story, so you have to cut them some slack.

I think Fran's advice can be applied to so many areas of life. When we are dealing with someone tricky at work, in the heat of road rage or on the receiving end of verbal abuse, we have no clue what is going on with the other person. We cannot visibly see their stress or what adversity they might be dealing with. It's not to excuse their behaviour or to negate our own feelings, but it can give us another angle from which to view the altercation.

Sadly, many in customer service roles are dehumanised and used to vent frustration and impatience. Having to deal with this on a daily basis can lead to disengagement in the role, built-up frustration or low self-esteem, depending on how you process stress. Over the years I have used disengagement as a coping mechanism. If I am finding a job stressful, I switch off and go into autopilot. I use my learned skill set to do the job but close off emotionally. I did this at times when I was working in radio in my twenties. If I felt overwhelmed at the relentless listener feedback, or shy and not in the mood to be putting myself on show, I would disengage. This may seem like a harmless coping mechanism to limit stress but over time there is a physical build-up and an emotional backlog that needs to be dealt with.

Little things to help with stress at work

If you feel you have a backlog of stress from the relationships in your life, whether work-related or not, do you have a way of releasing them? Next time you come home from work with stored stress in your body, try one of the below.

❀ **Punch a sofa or pillow on your bed.** Physically move the anger on.

❀ **Run or jog around the block.** Stomp out any stress.

❀ **Shake your body.** There is no particular way to do this: just shake all your body parts as animals do in the wild after they've been through a stressful encounter. Shake your body, legs, arms, head, hips and move the stress on.

❀ **Take long inhales and make a loud noise on the exhale.** A shout, moan or groan, to release the energy of stress.

❀ **Have a cold shower** and feel the stress release from your physical body.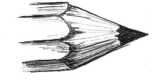

❀ **Daily journalling after work** can help decipher which emotions you're working with. It's a perfect way to cultivate self-awareness. It can create more space in your head as your thoughts become ordered and clear.

❀ **Create a daily care routine.** This will help you process every-day stress, which is essential for stopping long-term stress from manifesting in a physical manner. Daily, incremental stress can cause much bigger problems if not dealt with in the moment. It might not feel like it is doing much in the moment, but if we have a routine to help us rid ourselves from daily stress, long term we will feel a lot better.

CHANGE

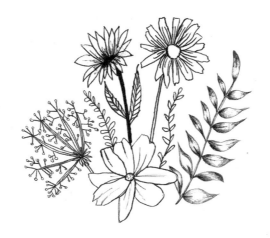

One of the only certainties in life is that we are going to experience change. The paradoxical nature of being certain of the uncertain can leave us feeling stressed and worried about change. It can also lead to excitement and growth, but we have to eliminate the fear of change to experience the positives. Nothing is permanent, so the ephemeral nature of life is a concept we have to navigate daily. Each day we wake up a day older, we experience different moods and weather, and we encounter different people, issues, challenges and experiences. How we navigate constant change is one of the factors that dictates how much stress we feel. Some of this will be informed by our upbringing and what was modelled to us in child- hood. Some of it will be due to the severity of change we experience. And some of it will be down to genetics. When I interviewed Robert Waldinger, who I have mentioned a few times already, he talked about the happiness baseline we all have. It is perhaps empowering to know that about 40 per cent of our happiness is in our control, and the rest is down to genetics and personality. We all know people who are glass-half-full types and those who are glass-half-empty. If you have a naturally positive disposition, you may navigate change more easily. If you are naturally a little more pessimistic, you may struggle when faced with change. Yet it is important to think back to that percentage. If we can control 40 per cent of our own happiness, that leaves quite a lot of room for improvement regarding how we navigate change.

As I have already outlined, change can be a huge trigger for stress, but we can also see it as something quite beautiful too. Recently my daughter left Year 2 at school and a teacher she was extremely fond of. As she climbed into bed after the last day of school, she wept and wept and explained that she didn't like the feeling of so much change. She would miss her teacher and she was also very scared and stressed about the changes she would experience in Year 3. We sat and talked about it for a good couple of hours and eventually got to a good place. I used the example of nature and how change is essential for growth and newness. Nothing in nature stays the same. Each season is a nod for us to notice life's ever-changing cycles. The small snowdrops pushing through the hardened winter ground, the amber leaves dropping from autumnal branches, the completely bare trees through winter. It's one constant cycle of change. If we want to grow, we must experience change. When things aren't moving and changing, we get stagnant. Change can be tough, but it can also be the making of us all.

The changes we experience daily will play out from the macro to the micro. Huge global events will mentally affect most of us and cause us to confront our beliefs and perspectives, as well as ignite empathy. Or if we lose someone, we will be forced kicking and screaming into a period of immense change. The micro-moments of change are more intimate and subtle, such as personal growth, breaking habits and forming new opinions.

In some ways, with age I have become better at dealing with change, yet I have paradoxically become fixated on routine and the safety within it. Now, in my forties, I'm perhaps better equipped to understand how my own moods are cyclical and am more accepting that nothing stays the same. I am better at adapting to new people and work challenges from years of practice. But, in other areas of my life I have become more rigid, like an old gnarly tree that stays put come rain or shine. I don't like surprises anymore, or spontaneity. I want plans, written lists, boundaries in place, so I can feel safe. I'm still very much a work in progress when it comes to mental flexibility and adapting to change. I think most of us experience moments where we fear change, but also moments where we are utterly stuck, both of which cause stress. When we are happy, we feel scared it'll leave us. When we are struggling, we can't see the opportunities to make changes.

I'm curious as to how we can create healthy routine that supports good habits yet allows room for spontaneity and growth. I believe if we find this balance and have a good relationship with change, we'll be better equipped to deal with unwanted changes and less inclined to feel stuck.

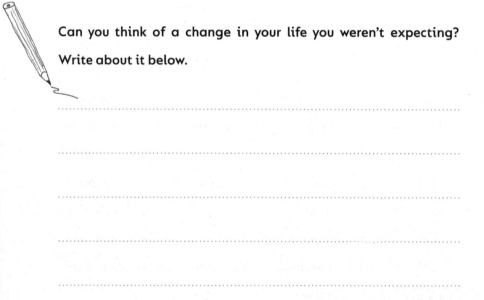

Can you think of a change in your life you weren't expecting? Write about it below.

How did you navigate this change? Chances are you're still in one piece and have built up resilience from experiencing it. What did you learn from this time of change?

....

....

....

....

Even if you were floored by this particular change, there is still time and room for growth and recovery. Often, when something challenging from the past still affects us, we get very used to the feelings of fear, sadness and stress. They become our new normal, even if underlying, and we get used to how they might be controlling portions of our lives. To start healing from such events it's important to be willing. We cannot repair without the will to do so. That healing might be cultivating a level of acceptance about experiences you have faced, or a willingness and desire to feel happier. If there isn't a will, there isn't a way.

STUCK/UNSTUCK

If we are unwilling to make changes or refuse to look at ones that are ongoing around us, we can feel stressed and stuck. Stagnation can cause lethargy, apathy, confusion and physical tension.

Recently I found myself feeling stuck in a cycle of poor sleep. Not only did I feel stressed from worrying that I wouldn't sleep each night, and stressed that the lack of sleep would ruin the following day, I also felt extremely stressed that I was trapped in this cycle. I began dressing up the stagnancy as acceptance. I told myself that insomnia and anxiety around sleep was just the downside of working a lot. I convinced myself that nothing could be done, and I had to accept that some days I would feel shattered. I was stuck, because I wasn't inviting change into the equation. When I'm stuck, I tend to put off the one thing I know will help. It feels like too much effort to make changes. In this instance I piled on even more work and ignored the advice from my husband to practise some self-care. Essentially, it requires less effort to remain stuck, yet it doesn't benefit us in the long run. Last week, after a lot of encouragement from my husband, I reached out to a friend I know who specialises in this area. We went for a long walk around the park, and I talked through my anxieties and the stress I felt at being so stuck in this torturous cycle. He has since given me some pointers to consider in parts of my life that need tweaking. There was no instant fix, or one solution, but I have willingly invited change into the equation, which feels like progress.

Are you putting off making changes?

During my procrastination and reluctancy to make changes, it became clear that I was scared it would require more effort and energy than I had available.

What scares you about making this change?

I haven't yet fixed my sleep, but I have made small steps towards change by reaching out to my friend and going for that walk. It helped that he called me out on my procrastination and quizzed me about why I was putting it off.

What small steps could you take?

....

....

....

Conversely, we may need time out to rest and take heed of big life challenges before we make changes, so it's essential to decide whether we are procrastinating or simply having much-needed down time. Katherine May, the incredible author and speaker, recently came on to my *Happy Place* podcast and we discussed the notion of wintering. Katherine's book, *Wintering*, felt like a sigh of relief to read, and I know many share that sentiment. Wintering is our natural need to step back, restore, hibernate, get small and quiet and let everything fall to shit. Sometimes we need to let the wheels come off so we can gain clarity and take a break from our own busy lives.

Think back to the natural cycles at play in nature. Nothing blooms all year round. Do you feel the need to retreat and slow down, or are you stuck and putting off change?

....

....

....

....

If you are wintering, then be gentle with yourself. Treat yourself kindly and allow yourself the space and time to grieve, cry, be still and retreat. Katherine explains that when we truly allow ourselves to do so, we naturally move into a new phase. Trusting that the period of wintering will naturally evolve takes courage, but Katherine is encouraging us all the way.

Little things to help you get unstuck

❀ **Challenge yourself to move out of your comfort zone.** Walk or cycle to work instead of getting the tube/bus/car. Try something new for lunch. Chat to somebody at work or at the school gates that you haven't approached before. Proving to yourself that you are capable of change in small ways builds confidence to create even bigger change.

❀ **Set your alarm for 30 minutes earlier than usual.** Give yourself that time to write in a journal, make yourself a nice breakfast or read a book you love. Switching up your daily routine encourages change and offers up new perspectives.

❀ **Write a postcard to a friend you miss.** Reaching out to others when we feel stuck can be a real lifeline. Receiving a letter or postcard is so much more personal and exciting than just getting a text. You'll be surprised how well this goes down with your friend and how much joy it brings you.

❀ **Change up your nighttime routine.** If you usually watch TV, try an evening walk with a friend or neighbour. If you usually scroll social media in bed, try putting the phone down and swapping it for a positive book. Small changes like this help to show us that we can rely on ourselves. When we switch up habits and make positive changes, we learn to trust that we can show up for ourselves.

✽ **Get creative.** Creativity is my saviour when I feel stuck. Writing, drawing, poetry, and painting can quickly get me out of a funk. Don't aim for a masterpiece or perfect outcome; this is all about the experience of creating. Creativity can also be described as 'flow', as there is constant progression and movement. It is hard to be stuck when you are in flow. Maybe just pick up a pencil and see what flows out of you.

✽ **Get outside.** If I am experiencing writer's block, I have to down tools and get outside. Sometimes a short reprise of fresh air and a hit of colour from the greenery around me is enough of a reset to carry on in a positive direction. If you are feeling stuck in any capacity, a good walk outside in nature (if that's possible for you) can help clear the mind and boost energy levels. Have you been outside today?

These suggestions might feel very unrelated to the situation you feel stuck in, but these little things will incrementally prompt a new confidence in switching your life up. Facing the responsibility of making big changes can feel extremely daunting, so start little and see how it makes you feel.

A note on creativity

If you have a creative job, it is important to remember there will be good days and bad days. During the writing of this very book, I have had blissful days where my hands dance over the keys with ease and ideas pour out of me. I have also had days where I have written one paragraph and felt stuck and stressed. I feel so fortunate to have a creative job, yet I know the perils of that often unknown, unstable, and trepidatious on/off flow.

ACCEPTANCE

Throughout this book we have looked at the little things we can change when it comes to reducing stress, but there are of course things we cannot change. We might wish we could change those around us, the weather or others' opinions of us. When change is impossible, we have one choice when it comes to reducing stress, and that is to land on acceptance.

I am having to practise this right now, as the Happy Place Festival looms in eight days and I feel stressed out about the unpredictable weather of the UK. I desperately want everyone coming along to have the best time and to leave feeling refreshed and boosted. I can barely even write the word *rain* here as I'm so worried about tempting fate. I know I can't control the weather, or indeed how much people enjoy the festival. All I can do is know that as a team we have done all we can to ensure there is great access to brilliant talks, workshops and classes, and the rest is the unknown. Having acceptance of this is the only thing allowing me to sleep at night. (I can now say months later as I work on the edit of this book, that we had a yellow weather warning and extreme wind during the London Happy Place Festival, and do you know what? We coped.

Everyone had a great time and we as a team learned a lot. We grew from the experience and gained a lot of confidence along the way.)

What I have learned over the years and from those I have interviewed is that acceptance isn't simply defeat. Having acceptance is not giving up; it's a peaceful choice that reduces stress. Another word for giving up is surrender, which has a different feeling to it. Giving up is throwing our arms in the air and frustratedly puffing out our cheeks in defeat. Surrendering involves a calmer approach, where we have thoughtfully chosen to have acceptance. Landing on acceptance may not change the situation we find challenging or negate all difficult feelings, but it will most definitely dilute the stress we feel.

Can you land on acceptance with the parts of your life you cannot change? Write a little about how that makes you feel below.

change

Finding acceptance is not easy. It requires courage, effort and strength. I don't believe there are people out there who are better at acceptance than others. We all have the capabilities; we might just need some support along the way.

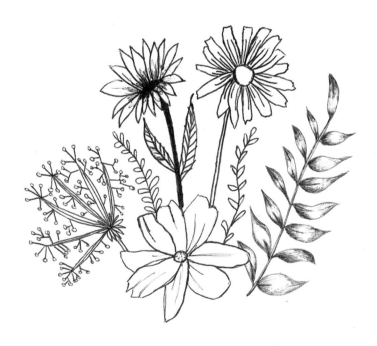

Little things to help with acceptance

❀ **Remember that it is hard.** Acceptance requires work, but it is not impossible.

❀ **Think about the stress caused by resistance.** What are you battling against and how much energy does it require? When we notice how much time and energy we are using on resisting parts of ourselves or parts of our lives we don't like or can't change, we can start to see the positives of having acceptance.

❀ **Express your emotions.** Talk to someone you trust or write down the feelings you're experiencing. If attempting acceptance makes you feel sad, or angry or frustrated, then admit it and talk about it. There is nothing wrong with feeling your feelings. We are humans and we are not here to get everything perfect. Owning our emotions allows us to move through them with more ease, rather than get stuck in them.

❀ **Be kind to yourself.** If you are finding it difficult to find acceptance, look at the challenges you face with self-compassion. These things take time and that is OK.

JOB LOSS/REDUNDANCY

Losing your job or deciding you need to make a big leap and leave your place of work is a change that's perhaps not so welcome. I, like many of you, have been sacked, and it always felt shitty and stressful. It usually leads to an intense period of self-doubt and questioning too. There is a funny unwritten rule in the world of TV: you can get sacked without even being told. I have turned on the TV to see other presenters hosting shows I once worked on, without having been officially told I'd been let go. I can almost laugh about it, as there is a bit of distance from that era of my life, but at the time it was stressful and humiliating. After a silent TV sacking I would usually end up spiralling and wondering if I would ever work again, questioning how I would support my family.

These are all very normal feelings, so if you have recently lost your job, just know that the pain is valid but also that it will not last forever.

Picking yourself back up after losing your job can be stressful because confidence is normally squashed in these moments. We assume we were sacked because we were dreadful and undeserving. It takes great resilience to try again.

Little things to help with confidence

❀ **Remember your skill set.** No one can take that from you. There is someone out there who needs someone exactly like you. Or could you use that skill set to start up your own endeavour?

❀ **Look at what can be learned from losing your job.** I learned that I can never be complacent about a job. It's taught me to be grateful each time I get work and has gifted me resilience, as I've had to think outside the box to forge forward with new projects.

❀ **If you have a job interview looming and feel terrified, stand like a gorilla.** My friend Justine taught me a technique that I still use today and have passed on to my children too. Stand with your legs hip width apart. Put your hands above your head in a V like a superhero. Pull your shoulders back, chin up, eyes alert. Give it some real physical gorilla energy, so walk into a room with purpose. Obviously drop your arms to the regular position before you walk into the room but feel the physical confidence of that pose and let it inform how you hold yourself in the room.

❋ **Know that every successful person out there has had huge knock-backs.** I can't think of a single successful person I've interviewed that hasn't experienced failure or rejection. Every author, sports personality, businessperson, actor: they've all been told *no* somewhere down the line. It's an essential part of the path to success.

❋ **Trying and failing is better than doing nothing at all.** Those who get knocked back have been brave enough to try in the first place, so commend yourself for doing so.

❋ **Create a wish list or vision board.** You may cringe at the thought, but it can be a really positive practice. You can try it now. On a piece of paper or in your journal, write about what you would really like to do, work-wise. Add some pictures if that helps create a visual too. You may not be able to move towards these goals immediately, but having these goals and dreams written down really does help bring them to life.

MOVING

When looking at short-term stress, moving home is up there as one of the most gruesome. Even a happy, planned move is stressful due to the admin, ever-changing timings and the practicalities of packing everything up, but also due to the emotional turmoil it creates. Home can be our sanctuary, away from work and the outside world, so moving can leave us feeling very exposed and vulnerable. We lose that sense of safety and comfort, so everything else in our life feels a little off-kilter. Jesse and I made the odd choice to move and get married in the same month. I have never felt so discombobulated by change. The practical organisation was immense, and it took me months afterwards to feel like there was any kind of order in my life.

Moving can also create stress as it can impact those we love. You might be moving away from relatives or friends or are nervous about moving to an area where you don't know anyone. You might also have children starting a new school and worry about how they will cope with that transition. One of my best mates recently moved from north London to Whitby Bay, where two of her sons had to start a new school. She felt stressed and worried about how they would deal with that change, but kids are often so much more versatile than us adults. Their brains are able to adapt more quickly than ours, all while cultivating resilience for change in the future. Luckily, both boys have already made loads of mates and have settled into the new area well.

The good news is the stress from moving is often temporary. It may feel all-consuming at the time, but it will pass as you settle into your new dwelling. If, like me, you find visual chaos very stress-ful, again remember that it is temporary. It may take months to get your new home in order, but you will get there.

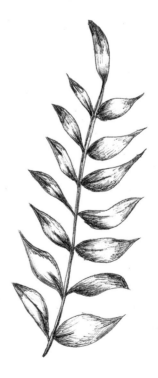

PREGNANCY AND NEWBORNS

The physical body goes through immense change when pregnant, again without much warning. We have a rough idea about how big our bellies will grow, but not many warn us about the hormone fluctuation, painful ribs, inability to sleep, giant nipples, heightened emotions and for some, like me, intense sickness for nine months.

My pregnancy with Honey was a rough, nauseous roller coaster where I hated all my favourite smells and on bad days couldn't even put the lights on. I scavenged online for how others coped and tried to stay in the moment as much as possible, to stop myself thinking about how many more months I had to endure the sickness. Every day and night felt like a nineties hangover aboard a ship riding a stormy sea. If Jesse made toast, I would have to run into the street to escape the smell. The scent of my car made me heave and our washing detergent made my toes curl. At times I felt incredibly stressed, as even doing the most basic task took Herculean effort. The positive that came from this period of change was being forced to listen to my body. There was no way I could ignore what it was telling me. It was shouting for me to rest more, take things at a slower pace and move through the day intuitively, rather than pushing through. None of that was particularly easy as I was working and had a two-year-old and two stepchildren to look after, but I took better care of myself because I had to. I must also point out the obvious, that it was worth every minute of excruciating sickness. If you feel stressed during pregnancy for whatever reason, know that it's completely normal. You are facing huge amounts of change and are having to adapt to it very quickly.

Having a newborn baby is one of the biggest life changes we can experience. It's a beautiful, often miraculous moment of change, but that doesn't mitigate the stress that we might feel too. It's a full-life one-eighty flip that we must get on board with instantly. Say goodbye to uninterrupted sleep, your social life, any downtime, oh and for some the function of your pelvic floor. I'm not really selling it here, but the point, among the heart-pounding euphoria of bringing new life into this world, is immense change. As we transition from no kids to one, or one kid to more, we have to constantly adapt and move with the changes at play. I used to naively wonder how a newborn baby could take up so much of someone's time. I assumed they just slept all day and occasionally fed. I soon realised that the cycle of napping and feeding was relentless and that the emotional concerns take up nearly all of your headspace.

It is completely normal to overly worry or feel anxious at this time. Checking your baby is still breathing while it's asleep is normal. Panicking that you're feeding them too much or too little is totally normal. Wondering if you're burping them correctly and feeling like you're winging it is 100 per cent normal. Hopefully, understanding that all of these feelings of worry are normal will reduce the stress of having a newborn, as so many others feel the same.

Little things to help reduce stress in the early days of parenting

❀ **Don't be afraid to ask for help.** Text your neighbour and ask if they could make you some soup you can pop in the freezer. Call your friend and ask if they could sit with the baby while you nap for an hour.

❀ **Do not be afraid to ask visitors to leave if you are exhausted.** You'll be inundated with lovely people wanting to meet your new family member, but the last thing you want in times of great change and exhaustion is Aunty Betty hanging around for five hours. All guests should know and understand the thirty-minute rule. Pop in, have a cuddle, then leave.

❀ **Don't worry about your home being a tip.** I wish I had worried less about this when my kids were newborns. I have inherited an insane level of house-proudness from my mother, and I found it hard to let that slip in the early days, but I would exhaust myself trying to keep on top of it all while looking after a new human. The dishes can wait.

❀ **Give yourself space.** Don't get too concerned that you haven't texted anyone back or called your friends. Everyone will understand. Go easy on yourself and take things at a pace you're comfortable with.

❀ **Don't suffer alone.** When you feel worried, stressed, or anxious about something relating to your baby, reach out to someone. Call a friend, text a relative and ask any questions you have. Online forums can be helpful, but be careful not to compare yourself to other parents or stories. Every pregnancy and baby are different.

❀ **If you need a good cry, have one.** It's perfectly normal, whether you are Mum or Dad, to feel huge surges of emotion. Crying helps release stress and move on energy, so have a good old weep and call someone you love if things feel too much.

❀ **Breast isn't always best.** If you are finding breastfeeding challenging, do not let anyone make you feel ashamed or like you are failing. Speak to your community nurse and see if they can help, but whatever you do, do not beat yourself up about it. You are doing brilliantly.

❀ **Find your family, your way.** Whether you have given birth, adopted, used a surrogate, are single and raising your child on your own, are in a same sex-marriage or are taking on someone else's children in a blended family, there is no one way to initiate family life. Do it your way, unapologetically.

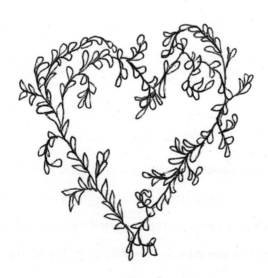

SAYING GOODBYE

Losing someone is one of the most stressful life experiences we can go through. Grief is layered and has the potential to stop time and change everything. If you have lost someone you love, you might feel you will never recover from that loss, or if your dynamic was complicated you might feel confused and anxious. There is no one way to experience grief. How we emotionally process loss is bespoke and individual.

Having interviewed many people about death and loss over the years, I often hear that in the West we are not particularly good at talking about death and are suppressed when it comes to grieving. Let's look at our cultural ideas about death initially. Many of us fear death, so we don't talk about it at all. In conversation we might use other phrases to skirt around the subject, such as *passed away*, *lost* or *passed over*. The word death feels too final, yet it is final, and we explicitly know this to be true.

When I interviewed Kelsey Parker about her late husband, Tom, who died of a brain tumour, she talked about the importance of using exact and plain language when talking to her children. She didn't want to use misleading phrases that would confuse the children further. She felt it would be damaging to tell her kids that their dad was up in heaven with the angels, so instead explained with care that their dad had died. I admire Kelsey hugely for having honest conversations about death. She is determined to show there is life after loss and is a beacon of light to others who have become widowed at a very young age.

I, like most, steer my thoughts from death. I believe we all have a natural reluctancy to stare it in the face, yet some don't have a choice. My dear friend Kris Hallenga has prompted conversations on death privately and publicly in documentaries, books and on social media. After a breast cancer diagnosis at the age of 23, she has lived with a terminal illness for the last 14 years. Kris has generously guided me towards the subject and has helped me become curious about it rather than terrified. Kris doesn't have the option, so over the years has committed herself to living her life fully while also acknowledging death. It's incredible to know that it's possible to think of death daily and live life fully. We might assume living with death in the wings creates a lethargy and sense of defeat, but if anything, it does the direct opposite.

Acknowledging death catalyses an awareness that we do not have time to waste, and Kris has lived in this way for much of her life.

Just last weekend she gifted her friends and family a spiritual experience and an opportunity to think about our own death and how we might approach it. Kris organised her own living funeral, naming it her FUNeral, as she wanted it to be a celebration of life. I was apprehensive in a completely self-centred way. I wasn't sure I could cope with saying goodbye to her while she was still alive, which doesn't make sense at all. Normally we wait until the person is no longer here to tell them how much they meant to us. Kris wasn't up for this, which is completely in line with how she has lived her life. She has never played by the rules. We cried as a gospel choir sang, we hugged each other when friends were giving heartfelt speeches, we laughed while comedians performed, we danced wildly to the DJ's music, we watched a glitter ball overhead throw flecks of light around Truro Cathedral. We celebrated life and we faced death, not just Kris's but our own. It was one of the best days of my life and has changed how I think about life and death. It's given me a new perspective on how I spend my days and has reduced the fear I have around death. If we can have healthy discussion about death, it won't take away the pain of someone leaving us, but it can help ease our fear of it, which subsequently dilutes the stress. If death is an off-limits conversation, it'll only build in its scariness and size.

Now let's look at grief and the stress that comes along with it. Again, in the West we are conservative with how we express our grief. We might have a period of mourning but then try to quickly get back to our everyday lives. We often feel we have little choice. Some will react to grief by suppressing emotions and numbing the pain. Some will experience long-term low mood or life-altering anxiety. Donna Lancaster, who is a grief expert, talks and writes a lot about unprocessed grief. If we do not allow ourselves to properly grieve, we get stuck in negative emotions, situations and mindsets. To grieve properly we need space, time and support. Another thing I've learned from Donna is that grief is a very physical process. You might experience a heaviness in your bones and pain or soreness in other areas. It's a full-body process of mind, spirit and physical body. Grieving is uncomfortable, back-breaking and often life-altering, but we have to let ourselves go through the process. Grief isn't linear, so there will be constantly changing stages of sorrow, maybe anger, devastation, moments of calm, then the cycle repeats.

Living with grief can be incredibly tough, so if you want more support don't be afraid to ask those around you for help. There are many great books on grief, such as Donna Lancaster's book *The Bridge*. We have also covered grief in many of the *Happy*

Place podcast episodes. I have chatted with Clover Stroud about losing her sister and how that grief felt extremely physical as well as deeply emotional. I discussed grief with Ashley Cain after the death of his daughter. He was courageous in exploring his very raw emotions with me and I will never forget this conversation. I also talked to Björn Natthiko Lindeblad one month before he died and we touched on grief, death and saying goodbye. It was the most powerful conversation I've ever had.

My husband lost his mum very suddenly when he was in his twenties. The grief was a sharp, shocking pain and the logistics stressful and burdensome. I hope his story offers you some solace and comfort.

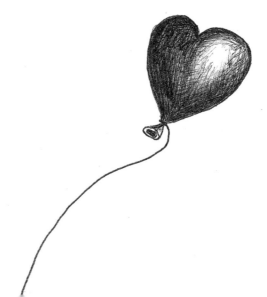

Interview with my husband, Jesse

Jesse, take me back to finding out about your mum's death and the feelings you experienced.

JW: My stepbrother Jamie rang, on 11 June. It was a warm and lovely day. I was living in Somerset at the time. I remember standing on the gravel driveway and picking up the phone, and looking down at the floor. Jamie then told me that the police had just visited him and then he delivered the news that my mum had died. It sounds odd to describe this, but you know when you're watching a film and they do that trick with a camera lens where it looks as though you're moving forwards and backwards simultaneously? It felt like that. I spiritually felt disconnected. I was aware that she had been partying a lot at the time: the month leading up to her death had been turbulent, as I knew she was drinking and using drugs. Part of me was worried, as she was 57, so I was scared about what the drugs could do. But I hadn't thought she would die. She died of a drug overdose. There are so many feelings involved, because you start to understand that the woman who created you is gone. You can never really get your head around that.

How did you cope with the stress of losing her?

I'm a recovering addict now, so at the time I dealt with it by drinking. Looking back, I have made peace with my coping mechanisms at the time. I was in total shock and found comfort in numbing the feelings by drinking. It's only recently, in the last ten years, that I have been sober and have been able to process the sorrow and stress and why I was running away so much. I now have better coping mechanisms when it comes to stress. I have picked up many tools like exercising regularly, talking to you (my wife) and meditating daily. I do a seven-minute online meditation every morning. I always try to step back and spot the patterns from the past. After having undergone the Hoffman Process, which is a week-long course in self-discovery and emotional healing, I understand the power of piecing together your childhood and viewing how you deal with stress, pain and adversity as an adult.

How did you deal with the stress of the paperwork and admin around losing your mum?

Luckily my uncles, my mum's three brothers, were there to help me, but it's a bit of a blur as I was in bad shape mentally. Together we sorted out the funeral arrangements, which felt so surreal. It was all so horrible, and because she died in shocking circumstances and I didn't know it was coming, I felt so shocked to be organising a funeral. The suddenness still makes me feel discombobulated. Some days I can even trick myself into thinking she is still here.

My dad's brother Art was really instrumental in support-ing me too and helping me through the whole process. I also had a young child, Arthur, to look after, so that gave me another focus. I also tried to concentrate on what music would be beautiful at the funeral and chose Coldplay's 'The Scientist', which really resonated. Concentrating on the power of music gave me a focus on the day.

Grief never entirely goes away, but the way I deal with the big emotions attached to grief is to see how many of my mums' traits live on in my four children, Arthur, Lola, Rex and

Honey. That always brings me great joy and is very healing.

Thank you so much, Jesse, for sharing that with us. I know it's never an easy story to tell. We talk about his mum, Krissy, all the time and have her trinkets and photos every-where in the house, so the kids feel she is still around.

MAKING DECISIONS

Think back to the last big decision you had to make. Remember the stress of having to make a decision that involved momentous change. We feel vast amounts of stress around decision-making because we feel the full weight of responsibility in these moments. We know deep down that our decisions will inform the trajectory of our lives. Anyone who grew up in the nineties, like me, will remember watching *Sliding Doors*, a film where Gwyneth Paltrow's character's life goes off down two totally different paths (with two different haircuts, one being a nineties crop that I'm still obsessed with) informed by whether or not she gets onto a certain carriage on the London Underground. I've been fascinated by these Sliding Doors moments ever since. When making decisions there is always the unknown. Even in the most calculated moments we have no real understanding of how things will turn out. Uncertainty can feel stressful, as we instinctively feel safer with the familiar.

Taking the stress out of decision-making

What was the last big decision you had to make?

....

....

....

How did you land on a conclusion?

....

....

....

Some of us will go with our gut, but in more complex decision-making, lists can help too. Looking at a pros and cons list is a basic approach to working out the answers to a decision, but still one I very much use to this day.

Have you got a decision to make now?

YES   NO

What is it?

....

....

Draw up a list of pros and cons for a little clarity on how you really feel.

PROS   CONS

....

....

....

....

....

....

....

change

Do you feel the conclusion from that list is the right one for you?
Do you instinctively feel relief or a spark of energy when landing
on that conclusion?

YES   NO

If not, why do you think that is?

....

....

....

Recently I was told that it's a good idea to only consult two people
when it comes to advice. Any more and our judgement starts to get
clouded, and the opinions become overwhelming. If you can pick
two trusted people who you know will be able to offer up impartial
and grounded advice, then stick to them. Don't feel tempted to ask
someone who you know could have a personal stake in the outcome
or is more emotionally driven when answering questions.

Who are your two chosen people?

1 ....

2 ....

Remember: either road taken will lead you to learn and grow. I'm not sure there is ever a firm wrong or right road to take. Even the biggest mistakes I have made, when walking down the wrong path, have led me to learn and at times gain resilience. If you make a wrong turn, it doesn't have to be life-defining. You can have regrets and wish you had done things differently, but try to do so alongside acceptance. Acceptance is the key to reducing stress. Life is messy, with multiple paths leading to different outcomes. Remember: if you take a wrong turn, it's not the end of the road.

GLOBAL MATTERS

As well as feeling the stress of change in our own day-to-day lives, there is constant change on a global level that can cause varying degrees of stress, whether it's the political landscape, climate and environmental issues, inflation or discrimination. There may be issues that you feel deeply passionate about, ones that ignite empathy, and some that make your blood boil.

We often feel stressed when we don't understand what is going on around us or feel powerless. The news is constantly rife with horrific and terrifying stories that can leave us feeling uneasy and unsure of what to do. If you already have stress in your everyday life, I think it's appropriate to give yourself a break from watching the news. If you are already overwhelmed, you won't have the capacity to take on the stress of negative news stories. If you are the sort of person who can sink into a low mood when the news is particularly sorrowful, I think it's worth remembering that the news is exclusively focused on the negatives. Yes, there are plenty of terrible things happening globally, but there are also magical moments of altruism, selfless individuals we may never meet and miracles happening.

In stressful times, seek out positive stories of hope and progress. I promise you they are out there.

If there are issues that cause you stress, one way to reduce it is to take action. If you feel sick to your stomach about animal cruelty, is there a local organisation you can help? If you don't agree with how some of the global brands operate, can you support local industries and small businesses? If you feel stressed about environmental issues, can you follow charities on social media that offer advice and ways to help with ocean clean-ups, climate change or soil preservation? I am constantly frustrated by the lack of support for individuals suffering with poor mental health or mental illness. I have interviewed countless people who feel hopeless, invisible, and unable to get the help they need. I also find myself in deep discussion about this very subject often, as people will email me or approach me in the street to explain their challenges. I try to channel as much of that frustration and stress as I can into my work with Happy Place. I have grand plans and it'll take time to instigate thorough progress, yet I am motivated to do better.

Finding others who care deeply about issues that cause you stress and pain can not only feel stress-relieving, but also empowering, so find likeminded people online or in real life. There is immense potential in alliance.

When speaking to the Earthrise gang – climate activists Jack and Finn Harries and filmmaker Alice Aedy – on my podcast a couple of years ago, Finn discussed activism burnout. Earthrise work tirelessly to create content and actively work in the climate change space. They've done some amazing work with raising awareness, through storytelling and on the ground with the community they have forged. At times, their work will be overshadowed by horrible statistics, environmental agreements being dismissed in government or a lack of support. This can all lead to burnout: a full-bodied exhaustion that signals retreat is needed.

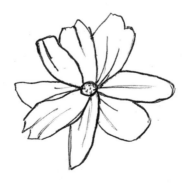

BURNOUT

What is it, and how is it any different to stress? Burnout is caused by accumulative stress without respite or rest. Here are the signs of burnout.

- ❀ physical exhaustion
- ❀ mental exhaustion
- ❀ emotional exhaustion
- ❀ creative exhaustion

You may experience symptoms like fatigue, insomnia, low mood, depression, headaches and changes in eating patterns. I have reached burnout on many occasions, as I tend to push myself to my limits. People-pleasing and aiming for perfection are also two lethal traits that have led me to burn out in the past. In these moments I feel overwhelmed, unable to cope and physically exhausted. I usually end up burned out because I don't believe I deserve rest.

I got pretty close to burnout in the middle of writing this book. I was juggling multiple other Happy Place projects alongside my home and family life and was being way too hard on myself. I could smell burnout on the horizon as I'd started to overthink everything.

This is a real warning sign for me. Mental overwhelm comes first, then physical fatigue and symptoms like tension in my tummy and headaches, followed by the symptoms of insomnia and irritable mood. Your warning signs of burnout might look different to mine.

List the symptoms you notice when you are heading towards burnout.

....

....

....

....

Burnout is hitting a wall. You have nothing left to give and might begin to experience apathy for the things you love as you don't have the energy and have a reduced capacity to cope with everyday life. We have to take heed of the signs of burnout, so we don't do more damage to ourselves physically and emotionally. You may wrestle with the idea and naturally push yourself too much, but you will be no use to anybody if you become sick or mentally unable to cope.

If you think you're experiencing burnout now, adjustments definitely need to be made. The first port of call is rest.

We are not good at rest in this country. It's almost been wiped from our dialogue. We see it as a dirty word, synonymous with laziness or weakness. It is in fact one of the most important factors when it comes to stress reduction. I am only just starting to realise its relevance when it comes to mitigating stress. Rest will look different to everyone, so find ways to calm your nervous system and reset emotionally that feel right to you. It might be one day not looking at your phone or laptop, a nap in the middle of the day, a weekend where you take it slow, a week off work, or early nights for a month. There is no right or wrong as long as you are slowing and calming down.

Little things to help with rest

❀ **Remember you deserve it.** It doesn't matter if others are working harder than you or have more on their plate. If you are burned out, you need rest.

❀ **Take moments throughout the day** to check in with how you feel mentally, emotionally and physically. Spotting where the tension lies gives us a gentle nudge to make changes to lessen it.

🌼 **Stop boasting about how much you do and have to do.** I'm not blaming you, but society. We have been brainwashed to emphasise how much we are doing and how little downtime we have as if it's a badge of honour. Life can of course be incredibly busy with work and family, but we have to find ways to celebrate rest and downtime too. If someone asks how you are, catch yourself if you begin with saying how much you have to do. Challenge the status quo by mentioning the time out you took for yourself or a future time when you are going to rest. It will encourage others to do the same.

🌼 **Enjoy the times of rest without guilt.** Sink into periods of downtime and remember that you are recharging like a battery so you can get back out there and get on with your wonderful life.

Burnout is physical as well as mental, so your body will need rest too, whether it's swapping running for walking, stretching every day or practising yoga nidra, which is a deep, still meditation. There are plenty of online meditations to choose from these days and we have many on our Happy Place app.

Somatic work that targets calming the body can be transformative in times of burnout, and although treatments can be expensive, if you can prioritise having a massage or reflexology you will feel instant results. Reflexology always works for me as it relaxes my physical body, helps with adrenal fatigue and feels delightful. When we are at burnout our adrenal glands really feel it. Our adrenals are small glands which sit on top of our kidneys and make the steroid hormones adrenaline and noradrenaline. These are hormones that help control heart rate and blood pressure. When we are at burn-out, these poor glands are working overtime, dishing out adrenaline non-stop. Treatments like reflexology can massively help with rebalancing the adrenal glands, as well as calming the whole nervous system. You can also ask your partner or best mate for a foot rub. You can google the points on the foot that target different areas of your body and work with those.

It might feel totally alien to you, but if you are at burnout you need to put YOU first. Even if it feels uncomfortable and you start to judge yourself or feel self-indulgent, there is no other option. If you carry on racing through life and pushing yourself, burnout could lead to other physical symptoms and illness. With burnout, rest is best. Believe me, you deserve it.

What does rest look like to you?

....

....

....

Next time you feel the urge to push through, could you try giving yourself time to rest? A mini-retreat for your body and brain? Next time you are willing to rest, try one of the below:

- ❀ A weighted blanket over your body on the sofa
- ❀ An online meditation
- ❀ A gentle walk outside in nature without digital distraction
- ❀ An hour away from any kind of screen
- ❀ Half an hour of silence
- ❀ A hot bath with gentle music playing
- ❀ A whole day of moving at half your usual speed
- ❀ An automated email response that lets others know you are not available

THE SOLUTIONS

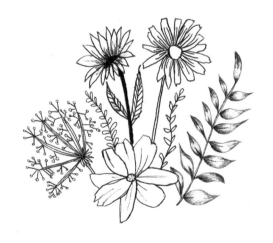

This book has been a real learning curve for me. Delving into the world of stress has awakened me to my own stress cycles, made me a lot more curious and unearthed a lot of great advice from others. It has also given me a lot to think about in terms of what causes us to feel stress and why, how our upbringing has a huge part to play in how we process stress, and how malleable and resilient we are when it comes to experiencing big life events. The interviews in this book have given me strength and inspiration, and also tools that I will take with me.

Here is a collation of my favourite tools and tips we have learned throughout the book to help with stress reduction.

❀ **Get out in nature.** Walk, run, meander, be in the great outdoors. Whether it's a local park, beach or a small green area near you, it all counts and will help with stress reduction.

❀ **If you are deep in stress, reach out and get support.** Whether it's talking to a mate, seeking professional help or leaning on a relative, don't think that you should suffer in your stress alone.

❀ **Make changes that work for you.** Set boundaries, tell people what you need, what you are capable of and what you are not. Leave toxic friendships, question your own beliefs about yourself, lose the negative inner chat, do more of what makes you happy.

❀ **Laugh more.** Watch funny films, hang out with people who make you howl regularly, find the humour in the embarrass-ing and cringey moments, tell stories to make others laugh. It's infectious.

❀ **Move your body.** Do this in a way that suits you and works with your body, not against it. Whether it's dancing, walking, body shaking to relieve trauma, yoga or otherwise, make sure you move your body with respect and care. It doesn't need to be punished or more stressed out than it already is.

❀ **Maintain a balanced diet.** Check how much caffeine and sugar you are consuming and make sure you are filling your plate with wholefoods instead of processed. Treat your body kindly and reach for snacks that will energise you rather than leave you in a slump.

❀ **Rest when you need to.** Do not push through and torture your mind and body with more tasks when you are exhausted. Pushing through can lead to burnout and serious physical consequences. Less screen time and distraction is key when it comes to proper, complete rest.

❀ **Try meditation or breathwork.** These will help you to slow down the nervous system. There are so many online practices you could try for free to help move you through stressful situations and to tell your body that everything is OK. If your body starts to get the signal that it's OK to relax, the brain eventually catches up too.

❀ **If you find yourself stuck in a rut, try something new.** Challenging yourself with new hobbies or tasks is a wonderful way to instil self-confidence and joy. More joy equals less stress.

❀ **Watch what you watch.** Ensure you are mindful of what you are watching, listening to and reading. Curate your media intake so that it's positive, inspiring and relaxing. Violent TV shows, shocking news stories and stressful articles are not going to help you when it comes to feeling calm and measured.

❃ **Listen to other people's stories.** This is not to fall into the trap of comparative suffering, which could lead to you not honouring your own story or pain, but to challenge your perspective and hear how other people have struggled and coped.

❃ **Release your emotions when they show up.** Don't suppress joy, or anger, or sorrow. If it is there, let it out by laughing, crying, stomping, punching pillows, shouting or making other noise, singing, running or whatever feels like it will honour the emotion. Once we have fully honoured an emotion and let it move through us, we can let it go. When we suppress emotions, we feel inner physical tension and outward stress.

❃ **Try out somatic work.** Massage, reflexology and craniosacral therapy can all help to release tension. See if there is a local practitioner who you could visit.

❃ **Remember that everyone is going through something.** When we believe we are being treated unfairly we have to remember that the other person has their own pain, suffering and stress to contend with. As Fran the air steward mentioned, we really have no idea what is going on with other people.

❀ **Be kind to yourself.** When we are stressed, we often make bad choices that lead to more stress. Trust yourself. You know you better than anyone else. You have way more answers than you think. Be gentle with yourself. Treat yourself like you would your best friend. Go easy on yourself. You really do deserve it.

I hope that the tools, practices, moments of reflection and interviews in this book have helped in some way. I was wary of making huge promises at the start of this book, as I am with you on this journey to reducing stress. I don't always have all the answers myself and even when I do, I can neglect them and get lost in the drama of life. Yet through the work I've been doing personally and professionally over the last six-odd years it is clear to me that it's the little things that really help make huge positive shifts.

I also hope that my own anecdotes, and the discussions I've had with others, go some way towards normalising stress. Often, when we feel stressed, we assume it's because we are flawed or unable to cope, but it's the most normal response to the amazingly fast-paced world we live in. When stress tips into burnout or physical symptoms, we need to take note of what our bodies are telling us. Never ignore the signs of burnout or physical exhaustion.

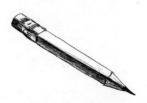

My hope is that you have doodled, written, scribbled and expressed many thoughts and ideas on these pages that have led to ideas, self-awareness and maybe even fresh solutions. I hope you feel empowered and have noticed how much possibility there is for positive change: even by looking back on your own musings you will see how you have so many of the answers already.

A stress-free world is perhaps optimistic and wishing for a stress-free life is not guaranteed. Life isn't meant to be neat, ordered and easy. There is beauty in the mess, growth in the chaos and resilience in the difficulty.

I asked the Happy Place community what helps them with stress reduction and here's what some of them had to say:

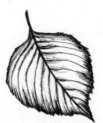

- ❀ Kate: Journalling
- ❀ Paddy: Breathwork
- ❀ Paula: Yoga
- ❀ Steph: Time alone
- ❀ Cat: Sleep or a cry
- ❀ Hannah: Therapy, books, a bath and cooking
- ❀ Em: CBT (cognitive behavioural therapy)
- ❀ Cally: A snuggle with a blanket
- ❀ Louise: Movement

- ❀ Rainbowstorm: Meditation, bubble baths, walking and listening to music
- ❀ Rob: Getting in the garden

My biggest learning throughout the process of writing this book is that our aim should not be to totally rid ourselves from stress, as that's often an unattainable goal; instead we should get through it. We can also practise responding to stress rather than simply reacting to it. The more self-awareness we have, the better chance we have of responding to stress rather than reacting to it. I hope you come back to this book often to journal, get curious and gain comfort. This book might be your reminder to check in with yourself weekly, monthly or even at the end of each year. Reducing stress takes practice and a daily discipline. There is no magic wand or route to an easy life. Everybody will face challenges of varying degrees and there is no exception to that. How we respond to stress is the part we have control over and is something we need to return to regularly. Keep looking at your priority pie chart, keep checking in with the section on boundaries to make sure you have some in place, keep noting down how often you are allowing yourself to rest. These small daily actions and thoughts will make a big impact on you and your stress levels. Remember: it's the little things.

ACKNOWLEDGEMENTS

This book would not have been possible without the generosity and wisdom from the experts and friends that feature in this book. This book helped to catalyse conversations I hadn't had before with people I know and love. Thank you so much Amanda Cotton, Abigail Tufano, Fran Blackburn, Liz MacCuish, Nicole Crentsil, Alice Liveing, Lin Cotton (aka Mum) and my husband, Jesse Wood. These conversations formed so much of the foundation of this book and its structure. A huge thank you to Dr Judson Brewer and Owen O'Kane for their expert opinions and advice too. Not only did I find those learnings incredibly interesting, but I have weaved them into my everyday life to help with my own stress levels.

I have written a fair few books now and, as well the process being incredibly joyful, there is of course stress too. The stress of worrying whether the book is good enough, the stress of looming deadlines, the stress of pushing my own limits to make sure I'm working to the highest level possible. I could not navigate that stress without the right team. Therefore, ginormous thanks is due to Lizzy Gray at Ebury who has been the most encouraging and calm guide throughout the writing of *Little Things*. At the point where I was ready to bin an earlier iteration of the manuscript, she kept me on the right path and reminded me of why I was doing it. Lizzy, as you move on to new adventures I wish you so much love and luck, and very little stress.

Thanks so much to Amanda Harris at YMU Group, who was the first person to trust in my writing abilities and helped ignite a whole new delicious literary path to walk down. I'm beyond grateful for your constant belief and encouragement. I'm in awe of how you juggle your demanding job and family life, and I have definitely learned a thing or two about stress management from our gentle conversations over coffee. You are incredible.

Sarah White at YMU Group, where do I start? Rather than keeping my thanks to the pages of this book I should email you a summary of my thanks daily, for all that you do. Your organisation, vision of the future, ability to listen to me moan about how I cannot cope regularly, and support in what I am trying to achieve is invaluable. It's a dream to have you by my side.

Matt Page at YMU Group, you're a legend. Thank you for helping me manage my workload and for always putting a smile on my face. Your natural calmness certainly helps level me out in stressful times and your one-liners are unbeatable. Thanks, Matt.

Thank you to Heike Schüssler for designing a cover that not only instantly calms me, but also illustrates exactly what this book is about. It's a beautiful cover that I believe will bring many people joy. Thank you to Evangeline Stanford, Jessica Anderson, Kate Latham, Leona Skene and Helena Caldon for their editorial eyes.

Rex and Honey, thank you for being the greatest teachers when it comes to stress management. Being a parent has given me the opportunity to practise patience, compassion and self-care in every way. In those moments where family life feels like total chaos, with lost school shoes, wet uniform still in the washing machine, arguments in the back of cars, refusal to eat vegetables, and so on, I don't always reach for the calm or sensible response, but I have plenty of opportunities to try again the very next day. I know I don't always get it right, but I am always giving it my best shot. You're the lights of my life and I will never stop kissing your gorgeous faces and sniffing your hair. Yes, Rex, even yours as you near teen-hood.

Arthur and Lola, thanks for being the coolest stepkids ever. I love our mad, messy family, and it's been a total joy to watch you both grow into adults and follow your instincts in life.

Jesse, thank you for dealing with me when I am very stressed indeed. Like most spouses, you get the brunt of it when I'm tired, coasting towards total burnout and in mega-bitch mode. Your acceptance of my inability to cope in certain situations and your ever calming words have got me through some pretty testing times, and I am forever grateful for that. I also know I don't say it out loud enough, so THANK YOU.

Thanks to my mum, dad and brother Jamie for your constant love. Mum, I'm so glad we chatted about stress for this project, and Dad, I'm so grateful for your constant calmness and navigation of stress with a cool and breezy approach. Love you all so much.

I guess I probably owe an uncomfortable thank you to everyone who has caused me great stress over the years. The individuals who have pressed my buttons, crossed my boundaries, called me names on social media and screwed me over at work, thank you. Thank you for helping me to learn and grow, and get curious about who I am and how I am built. I can't say it's been fun, but I know it's been essential.

My last thanks goes to you. Thank you for giving this book a go, it really means the world to me. I love writing books so much. The joy I get from delving into big subjects and writing freely about things I am passionate about will forever be a novelty and one that gives me great pleasure. I really hope this book helps. Thank you.

ABOUT THE AUTHOR

Mental health advocate, bestselling author, long-standing broad-caster, and founder and creator of the Happy Place brand, Fearne Cotton has been thoughtfully curating and building her Happy Place community since 2017.

Born out of sharing her own experiences with happiness, and publishing her *Sunday Times* bestseller *Happy* in 2017, the brand has evolved and translated into Fearne's award-winning podcast *Happy Place* (with over 105m downloads), the annual Happy Place Festival, which launched in 2019, the book imprint Happy Place Books in 2021, the Happy Place app in 2022, and the most recent addition to her portfolio, her Sky Kids animation show *My Friend Misty*, which was released in 2023. Fearne's previous book, *Bigger Than Us*, which published in January 2023, was another *Sunday Times* bestseller and further cemented Fearne's position as a celebrated author, with her books available in 12 different languages around the world.

Fearne is innately passionate about driving forward the notion of a relatable, straightforward and inclusive approach to self-care, and through her work with Happy Place has actively opened up, encour-aged and demystified the wider conversation around mental health.

Fearne is a mother of two, and stepmother of two, and is an active supporter for a range of charities, including mental health charity *Mind*, *The Prince's Trust* and *Coppafeel!*, the latter of which she curates the charity's music festival, Festifeel. Fearne is a supporter of the Princess of Wales #ShapingUs early childhood campaign, aiming to raise awareness of the vital role our early years play in shaping the rest of our lives.